The Three Stages of a Physician's Career:

Navigating from Training to Beyond Retirement

EDITED BY:

NEIL H. BAUM, MD
JOEL M. BLAU, CFP®
PETER S. MOSKOWITZ, MD
RONALD J. PAPROCKI, CFP®, JD

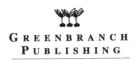

GREENBRANCH
PUBLISHING

PO Box 208
Phoenix, MD 21131
Phone: (800) 933-3711
Fax: (410) 329-1510
Email: info@greenbranch.com
Websites: www.greenbranch.com, www.mpmnetwork.com, www.soundpractice.net

No patent liability is assumed with respect to the use of the information contained herein. Although every precaution has been taken in the preparation of this book, the publisher and the authors assume no responsibility for errors or omissions. Nor is any liability assumed from damages resulting from the use of the information contained herein. For information, Greenbranch Publishing, PO Box 208, Phoenix, MD 21131.

This book includes representations of the author's personal experiences and do not reflect actual patients or medical situations.

This book is not intended as a substitute for the medical advice of physicians. The reader should regularly consult a physician in matters relating to his/her health and particularly with respect to any symptoms that may require diagnosis or medical attention.

The strategies contained herein may not be suitable for every situation. This publication is designed to provide general medical practice management information and is sold with the understanding that neither the author nor the publisher is engaged in rendering legal, accounting, ethical, or clinical advice. If legal or other expert advice is required, the services of a competent professional person should be sought.

CPT™® is a registered trademark of the American Medical Association.

Greenbranch Publishing books are available at special quantity discounts for bulk purchases as premiums, fund-raising, or educational use. info@greenbranch.com or (800) 933-3711.

13   8 7 6 5 4 3 2 1

Copyedited, typeset, and printed in the United States of America

PUBLISHER
Nancy Collins

EDITORIAL ASSISTANT
Jennifer Weiss

BOOK DESIGN
Laura Carter
Carter Publishing Studio
www.carterpublishingstudio.com

COPYEDITOR
Pat George

INDEX
Robert Saigh

TABLE OF CONTENTS

DEDICATION

Neil H. Baum, MD

This book has been made possible by the hard work and dedication of my co-authors, my family, and my medical colleagues. I would also like to thank my wife, Linda, and my three children, who are my inspiration and my greatest source of pride.

Joel Blau, CFP®

I dedicate my work on this book to the wonderful additions to our growing family: daughter-in-law Diana, son-in-law Brad, and grandsons Noam and Eli. I also want to thank the team at MEDIQUS for all of their assistance with not just the book, but also the contributions they make every day for the betterment of those who dedicate their lives to helping others.

Peter S. Moskowitz, MD

I dedicate this book to my wife, Susan, for her support and encouragement, to my co-authors for their boundless energy, wisdom, and unconditional friendship, and to the hundreds of practicing physicians who, as clients of my career and life coaching practice over the years, have informed my understanding and approach to the career management issues of physicians. It is through the candid sharing of their career and life stories that the wisdom contained in this book evolved.

Ronald J. Paprocki, CFP®, JD

I am grateful for so many of the individuals who helped me through the years, allowing me to enjoy a wonderful career and fantastic family. My wife, Joyce, deserves a special thank you for her never-ending support and commitment to our lives together. My sons have also been remarkable, serving as a source of joy and pride for our entire family. Finally, a special thank you to the entire team at MEDIQUS, who provide the environment to make my contribution possible.

ABOUT THE AUTHORS

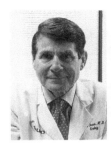 **Neil H. Baum, MD,** is a practicing physician in New Orleans, LA, and is a Professor of Clinical Urology at Tulane Medical School. He is the author of seven books, including *The Complete Business Guide to a Successful Medical Practice and Marketing Your Clinical Practice: Ethically, Effectively, Economically.* Contact him at doctorwhiz@gmail.com.

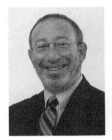 **Peter S. Moskowitz, MD,** is a nationally recognized authority on physician career management, speaker, workshop facilitator, and author. He is the Executive Director of the Center for Professional & Personal Renewal in Palo Alto, CA, providing career transition and life coaching for physicians nationwide. He is co-author of *Medical Practice Divorce*, a primer devoted to the topic of medical practice transitions, published by the American Medical Association Press. A pediatric radiologist by clinical training, Dr. Moskowitz brings to his coaching work over four decades of experience in both the academic and private sectors of American healthcare. He is currently Clinical Professor of Radiology, Emeritus, at Stanford University School of Medicine and at Lucile Packard Children's Hospital at Stanford. Contact him at www.cppr.com

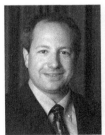 **Joel M. Blau, CFP®,** is President of MEDIQUS Asset Advisors, Inc. Prior to co-founding the firm, Mr. Blau was Vice President and Senior Financial Counselor for AMA Investment Advisers, L.P. Mr. Blau leads MEDIQUS's Institutional Services and has extensive experience analyzing and designing financial plans for healthcare professionals and medical organizations. He is an expert in not-for-profit investment management, wealth preservation through estate tax planning, retirement, investment, and insurance planning. He is the co-author of *The Prescription for Financial Health: An Authoritative Guide for Physicians, 2nd Edition,* published by Greenbranch Publishing. Contact him at blau@mediqus.com.

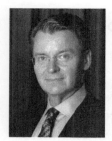 **Ronald J. Paprocki, JD, CFP®, CHBC,** is Chief Executive Officer of MEDIQUS Asset Advisors, Inc. Before co-founding MEDIQUS in 1996, Mr. Paprocki was Vice President of AMA Investment Advisers, L.P. Mr. Paprocki is responsible for the wealth management and the retirement plan services provided by MEDIQUS, which include the analysis and design of individual financial strategies for healthcare professionals, closely held business owners, and high-level executives. In addition, he is also responsible for the retirement plan services provided by the firm, which includes plan design, investment selection, and participant education. A Certified Financial Planner™ certificant, Certified Healthcare Business Consultant (CHBC), and Registered Securities Principal, Mr. Paprocki earned his law degree from DePaul University College of Law and his bachelor's degree from Knox College. He is the co-author of *The Prescription for Financial Health: An Authoritative Guide for Physicians, 2nd Edition*, published by Greenbranch Publishing. Contact him at paprocki@mediqus.com.

ABOUT THE CONTRIBUTORS

Randy Bauman is CEO of Delta Health Care, a healthcare consulting firm based in Nashville. He has over 30 years of experience in advising physician groups and hospitals on the business of physician practice, including practice valuations, mergers and acquisitions, group formations, and strategic planning. His first book, *Time to Sell? Guide to Selling a Physician Practice*, was published by Greenbranch Publishing in a third edition in 2016. His second book, *Choosing Autonomy—The Physician's Guide to Returning to Private Practice*, was published by Greenbranch in 2016. He is a frequent speaker to healthcare organizations.

Keith C. Borglum, CHBC, CBB, is a Certified Healthcare Business Consultant, private practice management consultant, and a multi-state licensed and certified practice business broker and appraiser, working nationally from his base in Sonoma, California, at MedicalPracticeManagement.com. He has been on the faculties and boards of directors for medical and business associations for many years, teaching physicians, CPAs, bankers, attorneys, and other consultants about the business side of private medical practice.

Neil Gesundheit, MD, MPH, is an endocrinologist and professor of medicine at the Stanford University School of Medicine. He has been the associate dean for academic advising at Stanford since 2006, and during this time has been the leader of the faculty group that has guided more than 1,000 Stanford students entering residency. He developed a practical algorithm to choosing a career in medicine, outlined in Chapter 2 of this book.

Thomas Shapira, Esq. advises clients on transactional and regulatory healthcare matters and represents numerous physician groups with respect to the formation and/or consolidation of medical practices, physician practice sales, and acquisitions. He has worked with healthcare providers to address numerous operational issues, including the creation of exclusive provider arrangements, hospital/physician joint ventures, and preparation of physician employment, compensation, and governance agreements, as well as managed care provider agreements and the establishment of ancillary services/facilities, including office-based laboratories.

Introduction

Neil H. Baum, MD

EVERY LIVING ORGANISM HAS A LIFE CYCLE—a series of stages it passes through from birth, through maturation, until death. Physicians, as human beings, go through this life cycle and, in a sense, so do their careers. This book chronicles the various stages of a physician's career, from the time he or she enters practice, through the development and maturation of the physician and his or her practice, and into the "golden years," as the physician contemplates retirement and eventually leaves the field of medicine.

THE EARLY-CAREER PHYSICIAN

We can liken the early-career physician's entry into the field as the beginning of his or her career life cycle—its birth. Early-career physicians are defined here as physicians in training (medical students, interns, residents, and fellows), physicians who recently started their practices, and physicians who have been in practice for fewer than 10 years.

Without a doubt, the most important career decision that medical students face is whether to specialize or have a career in primary care. Their studies and experiences in medical school can help them make that decision. However, they do not receive any information about the cyclical nature of medical careers and how to navigate the cycles successfully. The first two chapters of this book provide a narrative about the phases of the career cycle and the types of career transitions that flow from that cycle, along with a detailed strategy to guide medical students through the decision process when selecting a field of focus within medicine.

One of the first concerns of every graduate of medical school, a training program, or a fellowship, is whether to join a group and participate in a fee-for-service compensation model or become an employed physician and receive a salary and perhaps a bonus based on production.

The essential aspects of landing that first job are discussed in detail in Chapter 3. They are followed up in subsequent chapters with detailed and critical information about physician employment agreements, legal and financial priorities, and professional and personal finances—all areas that the medical school curriculum does not cover.

Beginning practice, whether as an employed physician, as part of a multi-specialty group practice, in a single-specialty group practice, or in solo practice, can be a daunting and stressful experience. The day you enter practice and are responsible for the clinical decisions you make, is the day you leave the womb of the training program and the day you really become a physician.

For the most part, young physicians or newly minted doctors receive no training or have first-hand knowledge on what to expect when they enter the world of real medicine. It usually takes months for new physicians to become acclimated and comfortable in their new practice surroundings. The pressure and responsibility can be hard to handle. It should come as no surprise that young physicians have a high rate of divorce, substance abuse, and even suicide.

My first piece of advice is to study the first six chapters of this book so you can lay the basic foundation for your practice. Then focus on being mentally prepared for your launch into a career in medicine.

As a healer, it's natural to become involved with and have compassion for your patients, but I suggest that you develop a modicum of personal detachment. To maintain your sanity and your objective ability to care for the patient and to make good decisions on behalf of the patient, you should keep some distance or least a psychological arm's length from the patient.

This is a difficult skill to do. Indeed, there is a fine line between compassion and detachment. It can be psychologically taxing to find that fine line between caring about a patient's well-being and health, then suppressing your innate sympathy for the suffering of a fellow human being—pain you may be personally inflicting.[1]

I am not suggesting that you be cold, distant, and uncaring as a physician. You can be concerned, a good listener, and attentive to your patients' needs without becoming involved in the periphery of their personal and private lives.

I also suggest that young physicians find a mentor in the community where they start their practice. New physicians often feel like fish out of water; they need help acclimating to their new role. Usually it is not the clinical decisions that provide so much angst, as it is the blending in with the community and the practice that are often the greatest challenges. Perhaps one of the best ways to make the transition from training to practice is to find a mentor who will take you by the hand and lead you so you can avoid the many pitfalls of medical practice.

Look around and you likely will find an older, established physician whom you admire not only for their clinical skills but also their stature and reputation in the community. A mentor probably should not be someone in your practice or even in the same specialty. Most mentors are honored to be asked to help a younger physician and are delighted to share their wisdom. A good mentor not only leads and encourages you but also tells you the honest truth.

If you don't know someone personally—or even if you do, do your homework before approaching a leading physician in the community to be your mentor. Go to the Internet and learn as much as you can about your potential mentor: his or her accomplishments, achievements, community activities, family life.

Call and ask for an appointment with your potential mentor and be available any time that is convenient for him or her. When you meet, request his or her mentorship and share your expectations with regard to speaking/meeting on a regular basis and more frequently in the event of pressing issues that require immediate attention. Follow up with a handwritten thank-you note whether your candidate accepts your invitation or not.

The best way to say thank you to a mentor is to become a physician that makes the mentor proud and then pay it forward and become a mentor to others who follow you.

THE MID-CAREER PHYSICIAN

A mid-career physician is defined here as the doctor who has been in practice for 10–20 years or is age 60. These physicians have belonged to solo or small-group practices, have used paper charts, and may be out of their comfort zone when trying to use new technology in the office setting.

It is the mid-career physician who complains that mounting paperwork is keeping them from spending enough time with patients. In The Practice Profitability Index, the percentage of physicians who spend more than one day per week on paperwork increased from 58% in 2013 to 70% in 2014. Nearly one-quarter (23 percent) spend more than 40 percent of their time on administration, up from 15 percent in 2013.[2]

This trend of more paperwork is eroding physicians' on-the-job happiness. Most physicians truly enjoy spending time with patients and anything that takes doctors away from eyeball-to -eyeball time with patients subtracts from their enjoyment of the practice of medicine.

Another concern that is affecting mid-career physicians that was not an issue when they started their practices is the requirement to obtain prior authorizations for procedures, tests, and for prescribing medications. The average physician spends 20 hours per week on prior authorization activities. That's 868.4 million hours per year on prior authorization at a cost of $69 billion each year to interact with insurance plans.[3] Prior authorizations represent a negative aspect of providing healthcare that probably affects the care that physicians provide their patients.

The Cost of Running a Practice

Physicians who are not employed by large groups or hospitals will have to contend with the rising overhead costs, which will be a problem to be solved by mid-career physicians.

There is no denying the cost of running a practice is going up. With reimbursements declining, rising overhead has cut into profits for the practice. Perhaps it shouldn't be surprising that in this constantly changing ecosystem, more practices are struggling to maintain financial homeostasis. An August 2013 survey by the Medical Group Management Association (MGMA) showed that the cost of running a practice had increased twice as fast as the consumer price index during the previous 11 years.[4] The mid-career physician will be challenged to rein in overhead costs for his or her practice.

Contemporary practices are seeing increasing rent, increasing rates for malpractice insurance and for directors' and officers' liability coverage, and higher health insurance costs for their employees.

IT costs are impacting the bottom line. The cost of the hardware and software for a practice management system and an electronic medical record continues to increase. There are costly maintenance contracts as well as expensive upgrades to stay compliant with HIPAA and quality measures. Most physicians (85%) have transitioned to electronic health records to comply with meaningful use, according to The Physicians Foundation survey, compared with 69% in 2012. This isn't cheap. The average five-year total cost of an in-office system electronic medical records is $48,000. For a cloud-based system, it's $58,000. These costs are in addition to the loss of productivity that many physicians experience during the implementation process.[5]

Shifting from Fee-for-Service to Pay-for-Performance

A new trend that will impact mid-career physicians is the measurement and then the compensation for patient satisfaction. This trend will also coincide with the shift from fee-for-service to a pay-for-performance compensation model. Now the experience of the patient, the appropriateness of care provided, and the outcomes will be measured and the doctors' compensation will be reflected by those data metrics.

Of course, these measurements will require expensive and sophisticated computer systems to record those data points. The take home message is that the mid-career physician will need to adopt to a movement from volume to value. Failure to implement these quality measures may result in financial penalties for not reporting Physician Quality Reporting System (PQRS) data to the Centers for Medicare and Medicaid Services (CMS). Beginning in 2015, practices that had not reported PQRS data in 2013 will be penalized 1.5% in their Medicare reimbursements.

Independence or Employment

The result of so many changes will certainly influence a mid-career doctor's decision to remain independent or to opt for employment by a hospital or other large group entity.

Many mid-career physicians will try to resist the pressures to give up independent practice. For some physicians, joining a large hospital system offers a safe harbor from the rising administrative burdens of staying independent and from competitive pressures that can drive a small practice into collapse. But joining a hospital system is not a panacea for the challenges facing the mid-career physician. This will be covered in Chapter 3.

Caring for Patients

One of the biggest challenges for the mid-career physician is that physicians' decisions regarding patient care are going to be monitored. Physicians are going to receive a performance grade card, so to protect their livelihood they tend to modify their practice patterns, to be more productive and improve their scores. The trend is going to be a movement to a metrics-centered business, rather than a patient-centered profession.

Patient satisfaction will be of paramount importance. No longer can the mid-career physician take a history, make a diagnosis, write a prescription and tap the patient on the back and see the patient in two weeks. Now, the doctor will have to be sure that all the patients' questions are answered before they leave the exam room.

Another element of patient satisfaction will require patient education. For example, patients can be asked at the time of their request for an appointment "What is the reason that you would like to see the doctor?" The receptionist or scheduler can lead the patients to the practice website and provide educational material on the topic of interest to the patients. Now the patients are educated before seeing the doctor.

The patient can also receive educational material at the time of visit, such as frequently asked questions about the medications that are prescribed. These educational materials are far more important and useful than the package insert that is included when patients picks up their prescriptions at the pharmacy.

Finally, the doctor and the practice can continue to interact with the patient after the patient leaves the practice. The patients' email addresses should be obtained at the time of their visits and the patients should receive a practice newsletter on a regular basis.

The ACA's Impact on Malpractice

The Affordable Care Act is going to add millions of Americans to the healthcare rolls. This will mean more patients, and many of these patients are going to require more healthcare services since they have been without healthcare for years or even decades.

As a way to avoid potential liability, some physicians report practicing defensive medicine. Erring on the side of caution, physicians order more diagnostic procedures than might be necessary to head off litigation.

THE LATE-CAREER PHYSICIAN

General McArthur once said, "Old soldiers never retire, they just fade away." Older physicians would like to stay connected to the practice of medicine, and if they have to fade away they have as a goal to leave with their reputation intact.

The retiring physician is usually in his or her 60s and is focused on winding down the practice by doing less and having less responsibility. Retiring is not easy and creates challenges for doctor and the practice. While many retiring physicians are on "auto pilot" and yearn for the good ol' days of autonomy, independence, and fee-for-service, the reasons that doctors are leaving include:

- Economic factors such as medical malpractice insurance, overhead, and electronic medical records;
- Healthcare reform;
- Burnout;
- Pursuing different career paths outside the practice of medicine;
- Lifestyle choice;
- Age 65+;
- Health reasons; and
- Financial ability to retire—the best reason of all.

Many doctors have a hard time knowing when it is time to call it quits. I know doctors who continue to practice into their 70s and 80s. Some continue to work until the day they die. Why is this? Many fear retirement, which represents an unknown future. They don't know what they are going to do for 40–50 hours a week when they stop practicing medicine.

I think that some doctors believe that it is somehow ignoble to leave the profession, that they would be abandoning their patients if they retired. If a doctor has provided care to the patient for decades and has cared for other family members, there will be an attachment that neither the doctor nor the patient wants to end.

Certainly, most doctors enjoy what they do, deriving a sense of satisfaction from their work. They take pride in their skills that have taken thousands of hours to hone and to master. Some enjoy the social status that comes from being a doctor and they worry that their social ranking will be gone when they retire. Some have matched their lifestyle to their income and think they can't do without the revenue. Some are hooked on the sense of accomplishment and euphoria that comes from opening a clogged artery in the middle of the night and saving a life, or ablating an arrhythmia and changing someone's life for the better.

One of the most difficult challenges facing the retiring physician is moving from a structured life that he or she has led for over four decades to an unstructured life where there are no meetings, deadlines, or calls to return.

As physicians, our lives are centered on structure; we are addicted to the clock. There are meetings, and patient appointment times, and starts times in the cath lab or operating room. There are calls from nurses and patients every day that vie for our immediate attention.

The challenge that most retiring doctors face is having so much unstructured time that they are bored. This requires balance between structured time and unstructured time that is necessary to provide stimulation without the requirement of responsibility.

These are just some of the reasons doctors are afraid to retire, or don't know how to do it. In Chapter 13 we discuss how to proactively prepare yourself for retirement, or "protirement." We suggest a plan of action for health, meaning and stimulation in retirement. Our goal is to help the retiring doctor transition from the practice of medicine to years when he or she can enjoy the well-deserved fruits of the labor of their medical career.

Every profession faces issues associated with leaving the profession and moving on to something else for which they have no training or skills. The accountant, the lawyer, the dentist, and even the young professional athlete has concerns about moving to the next phase of life that doesn't involve the skills and training that is required to be a professional. Like John Elway of the Denver Broncos, who retired after winning his second Super Bowl title, it is better to retire at or near the top of your game, rather than hanging on until your skills diminish and you have overstayed your welcome. Retire while you are still healthy and active enough to enjoy life. Don't wait until it is too late.

BOTTOM LINE

The three stages of a physician's career are predictable. It is not easy to become a doctor and it is not easy to move from one stage to another. This book is intended to help make those transitions easier and make the practice of medicine more enjoyable from the day you place the announcement of your entrance into clinical practice until the day you take down your shingle and ride off into the medical sunset.

References

1. Shadowfax. Dealing with the psychological stress of being a doctor. Kevinmd.com. Jan. 21, 2013. Available at: http://www.kevinmd.com/blog/2013/01/dealing-psychological-stress-doctor.html

2. Electronic Health Reporter. 2014 Practice Profitability Index: Physicians find declining practice profitability in the year ahead; Administrative burdens sharply increasing. Electronic Health Reporter. Available at: http://electronichealthreporter.com/2014-practice-profitability-index-physicians-find-declining-practice-profitability-in-the-year-ahead-administrative-burdens-sharply-increasing/

3. Bendix, J. The prior authorization predicament. Medical Economics, July 8, 2014. Available at: http://medicaleconomics.modernmedicine.com/medical-economics/content/tags/insurance-companies/prior-authorization-predicament?page=full

4. AAFP. Rising operating costs top list of medical practice concerns. AAFP. August 8, 2013. Available at: http://www.aafp.org/news/practice-professional-issues/20130808mgmasurvey.html

5. Terry K, Ritchie A, Marbury D, Smith L, Pofeldt E. Top 15 challenges facing physicians in 2015. Medical Economics. December 1, 2014. Available at: http://medicaleconomics.modernmedicine.com/medical-economics/news/top-15-challenges-facing-physicians-2015?page=full

The Early-Career Physician

CHAPTER 1

Understanding Modern Career Theory

Peter S. Moskowitz, MD

P HYSICIANS RAISED IN THE 1950s, '60s, and '70s grew up with a set of assumptions about life and work. The most important of these assumptions was that careers were linear—that the harder and longer one worked, the greater the rewards from work. This Linear Rule is no longer valid in today's rapidly evolving workplace. In its place is the Circular Rule, which stipulates that careers are cyclical over time and the phases of the cycle are predictable.

CAREER TRANSITION THEORY: THE CAREER CYCLE

To be more effective in the workplace and in managing their careers, physicians should understand this career cycle, which is illustrated by the Cycle of Renewal (Figure 1-1). The Cycle of Renewal is a conceptual representation of how careers and relationships change with time. Largely the work of Frederic Hudson,[1] the Cycle of Renewal includes four quadrants that represent career phases:

Phase I: Go For It
Phase Two: The Doldrums
Phase Three: Cocooning
Phase Four: Getting Ready

The following is a description of each phase, as seen through the lens of a practicing physician.[2]

PHASE 1: GO FOR IT

This is the first phase we enter when we've completed our training and education. It is the phase during which we land our first "real" jobs and are excited about our career and what it holds. It is a time of building our practice. We have all the new knowledge, are energetic, and love what we are doing. Physicians often buy their first home and have their children during this phase.

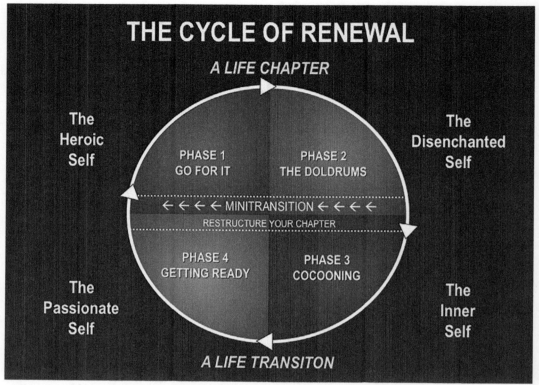

Figure 1-1. The Career Cycle (Reprinted with permission from the Hudson Institute of Coaching, www.hudsoninstitute.)

We are living the American dream and believe that it will go on like this forever—and no one tells us otherwise. However, for 95% of us, the bliss of the Go For It phase does not go on forever. Eventually we reach a plateau. Things begin to change for the worse and we slowly begin to move into Phase 2.

PHASE 2: THE DOLDRUMS

The Doldrums phase usually begins with a subtle shift in attitude. What used to be an exciting job starts to become dreary, dull, and boring. The partners we used to enjoy and find stimulating are beginning to become a pain in the rear. We no longer agree with the decisions and directions of our work partners. We lose interest in reading our medical journals. We find ourselves antsy with patients, lacking empathy, distracted. We get into conflicts with our co-workers and patients more often. We blame the system, hospital managers, and managed care.

We feel like victims, powerless to change the system. We long for things to return to the way they were in Phase I. We secretly feel guilty and depressed for having these feelings and are reluctant to discuss them with colleagues and friends. Or, we deny these thoughts and feelings as long as we can, preferring to suffer in silence.

Eventually we may begin to self-medicate with work, alcohol, prescription drugs, sex, gambling, or other unhealthy behaviors to escape the feeling of being trapped by our lifestyle and our own expectations and those of others.

Some stay stuck in this stage for many years. Others eventually "hit the wall" and experience a crisis of self-confidence and self-doubt that erupts into their work and relationships. We ease into Phase 3.

PHASE 3: COCOONING

Cocooning is a phase of low energy in which we reduce our commitments to career and devote an increasing amount of time to self-exploration. It is a time when we deliberately slow down and work less. It is a time for thinking and being, rather than doing. We spend time alone in quiet reflection.

For some, it may mean taking a sabbatical; for others, it may mean taking an extra day off each week, taking an extra hour each day at lunch and going for a long walk alone, or reading alone for an hour or two each day. Some physicians participate in psychotherapy or career coaching.

This is a time to reevaluate and decide what is truly important in our lives. What is our purpose? What are our values and passions? What is our calling? These are questions we may not have thought about since our college days. We have not taken the time to allow our life experience and personal growth to catch up with our vision of who we were in our 20s. For many of us, our values and purpose have shifted and left us out of synch with the values and expectations of our current workplace. As we explore and re-familiarize ourselves with who we have become, we slowly enter Phase 4.

PHASE 4: GETTING READY

Our self-assessment has uncovered past interests, hobbies, and passions that we had to abandon during the rigorous years of education and training. Perhaps they are things we had always intended to learn about, but ran out of time and energy. In Phase 4, we begin to explore them.

We take night classes at the local community college. We read books. We find that we have aptitudes we never knew we had. We re-engage with old interests, hobbies, and sports. We discover new talents, abilities, and passions. Some of these bring such joy that we want to do them more regularly. Some of these things may even open the door to potentially profitable new careers!

Intrigued, we begin to network with people who are doing those things as a career, learn how they got their breaks, what the outlook is for these careers, and how much money can be made—this is called informational interviewing. We make new commitments to move forward with those new dreams. This may require more education, perhaps a master's degree, a new residency, a new professional degree, or some form of professional certification training.

This career change fills up Phase 4. Eventually, we are retrained and acquire new skills and abilities. We begin a new career, a substantially different clinical career, non-clinical career, or a new career outside of healthcare. As we put that new training into action, we find ourselves back in Phase 1 again. But this time we're older, wiser, with new skills, and enjoying a career that is substantially different than the one we began many years earlier.

BACK TO THE BEGINNING

For most professionals, a trip around the periphery of the career cycle map takes a couple of years—although for some, the trip is shorter or longer. What is certain is that working with a career coach or career counselor will shorten the duration of your trip around the cycle to get back to Go For It.

There is the option of cutting across the career cycle, going directly from the Doldrums back to Go For It, in a move known as a mini-transition. Mini-transitions have one important advantage over full-career transitions: mini-transitions typically take six months or less. Mini-transitions are discussed in greater detail in Chapter 8.

Knowledge of the four phases of the career cycle, the direction of movement on the cycle, and the two types of transitions that evolve from cycle theory enable physicians seeking career change to manage their transition more effectively and with greater confidence. Using the career cycle map to your advantage, you will recognize when your career gets stuck in the Doldrums, and what to do to get unstuck by moving on to a mini-transition or a full-career transition. And, you won't even need Google Maps to get yourself back to Go For It!

References

1. Hudson, FM, and McLean, PD. Life Launch: A Passionate Guide to the Rest of Your Life. Santa Barbara, CA: The Hudson Institute Press; 1995.
2. Moskowitz, PS, Blau JM, Harris, SM, and Paprocki, RJ. Medical Practice Divorce: Successfully Managing a Medical Practice Breakup. Chicago: American Medical Association Press; 2001.

CHAPTER 2

A Primer for Choosing a Career in Medicine

Neil Gesundheit, MD, MPH

MEDICAL STUDENTS BEGIN THEIR MEDICAL STUDIES with diverse interests that developed from earlier life experiences and college coursework. Based on this prior background, some students seem to have decided on their field for post-graduate training from day one. For example, a student who completed an undergraduate degree in the neurosciences may bear the conviction that training in neurology or neurosurgery will provide the most fulfilling life path.

While it is important to prevent "premature closure"—the cognitive error of making a decision early, in this case a career decision, before sufficiently considering all alternatives—some students feel a true calling for a particular field and are laser-focused on making progress toward their career goal early in medical school.

Other students—the vast majority entering medical school—are uncertain about their trajectory and are eager to explore career possibilities. Choosing the "right" career, a career that aligns one's life and career goals, is an important decision. In fact, given that a medical career for most physicians spans from their mid-20s to late-60s, at least a 40-year timeframe, it is arguably the most important decision that a medical student can make.

During career planning, advisors often speak about a "good fit," meaning that the intellectual, physical, and lifestyle challenges of the field of clinical practice *fit* with the multidimensional aspirations of the student-physician. This chapter will provide a streamlined, practical algorithm, based on literature and methods that have been used successfully at the Stanford School of Medicine, for students who are choosing a medical career. The algorithm can also be used by physicians who are changing paths in mid-career.

FINDING YOUR PASSION: THE FOUNDATION FOR A MEDICAL CAREER

It is almost a cliché to speak about pursuing one's passions in medicine, but the reality of medical training—given its rigor and sacrifices—is that unless one is passionate about the chosen work, it is difficult to withstand the long hours, sleep deprivation, and decade of education and training required to gain the well-honed expertise of a skilled practitioner.

Having one's passion provide the motivational fuel needed for clinical training is not a new idea, nor is the idea confined to medicine. Steve Jobs, the computer technology pioneer, described in his 2005 Stanford commencement speech how he overcame adversity and turbulence in his work as a founding member of Apple Computer:

"I'm convinced that the only thing that kept me going was that I loved what I did. You've got to find what you love."

It is a love of the heart and how it works that keeps the cardiologist interested in improving the cardiac output of a patient in congestive heart failure at 3 a.m. It is the love of abdominal anatomy that motivates the surgeon to leave a family dinner to remove a ruptured spleen in the patient brought to hospital after an automobile accident.

It is therefore incumbent upon medical students, most of whom are attracted to medicine because of their aspiration to use science to improve human lives, to reflect on what aspects of clinical practice create the deep motivation that results in self-sacrifice and transcends time and remuneration. Conducting a personal inventory is often helpful in defining the field of practice that resonates with and nurtures this motivation.

MAKING THE *RIGHT FIT* FOR A MEDICAL CAREER

Students often benefit from conducting a personal inventory of their own abilities, motivations, and needs before they explore the characteristics and offerings of a field of clinical practice. Several personal inventory instruments are available to allow such a self-assessment (see the Careers in Medicine website from the American Association of Medical Colleges, www.aamc.org/cim). These self-assessment tools examine the following components:

1. Aptitude

Certain fields of practice require innate abilities that not all students possess. As an example, several years ago, my colleagues and I counseled a medical student who was interested in surgery, especially fine surgery that required the use of a stereoscopic surgical microscope. While he appeared to have excellent fine-motor skills, he suffered from amblyopia ("lazy" eye) because he had had strabismus as a child that was not corrected until high school. Because of his poor binocular vision, he lacked the basic ability to excel in microsurgery. We therefore counseled him against pursuing microsurgery.

In contrast, in the case of another student who had been successful in creating artwork and glass sculpture, we strongly endorsed her pursuit of surgery. She was keenly interested in oculofacial plastic surgery and seemed to have special hand-eye coordination and an artistic aptitude that would integrate itself nicely and be a strong asset in plastic surgery training.

2. Interest

Strong aptitude for a field of training must be complemented by strong interest. Students often become aware of their vastly different interests during the pre-clerkship curriculum. As an example, for some students, gross anatomy offers a fascinating glimpse inside the human body, whereas for others it is as exciting as the unveiling of a road map. Some students thrive on performing anatomical dissections, which allow them to demonstrate and exercise delicate, fine-motor skills; for others, gross anatomy dissections represent loathsome drudgery.

This divergence of student interest is also apparent in coursework in biochemistry, physiology, and pharmacology. Some students are intrigued by how a molecule can bind to a receptor, convey a signal, and mediate an important physiological activity. Other students find these molecular events remote and difficult to understand. These nearly visceral differences in students' interests are important to factor into the decision about which field of training creates the right fit.

3. Values and Work-Life Balance

A field of clinical training must reflect the values of the trainee and allow a continuation of activities that sustain these values. Values refer to the deep-rooted beliefs that dictate what kind of lifestyle one chooses and allows one to invest intellectual effort and time in pursuit of life objectives. These are some of the work-life balance considerations that we have encountered that reflect medical students' underlying values and shape their choices:

- How do I ensure that my job affords me time for community and volunteer work, teaching, public service, hobbies, artistic pursuits, spirituality?
- How do I maintain my professional standing while devoting sufficient time to creating and nourishing a family?
- For students aiming for academic medicine: How do I maintain and fund my research and scholarly activities? How do I plan to apportion my time between research, teaching, and patient care?
- For all students and practitioners: How do I maintain a healthy work-life balance?

Remuneration can also factor into the assessment of one's values and the desire for work-life balance because a highly remunerated field can increase the amount of time that a practitioner has available to pursue other interests. For example, an anesthesiologist may earn as much income in three work days in the operating room as a pediatrician does in five work days in the office (in addition to taking night call). By working only three days each week, the anesthesiologist can potentially engage in other activities consistent with his or her values, such as coaching a Little League team, serving on city council, volunteering in a local church/synagogue/mosque, or joining an art studio and creating new canvases.

It is difficult for medical students to predict in advance the specific work-life balance they seek; most students, however, have a general estimate of the proportion of time that they want to devote to work compared with other activities. This estimate should factor into these questions of work-life balance when choosing a field for clinical training.

4. People

Another important consideration for students choosing a field for clinical training is the people they will work with—their colleagues—and the people they will serve—their patients.

An early indication that a student is well-matched for a field of training is that the student feels "at home" with residents, staff, and attending physicians in the potential field of practice. Often, affinity for the people practicing in the discipline is lacking at the outset, but an attraction develops over time as the student becomes acculturated to the field. At other times, a student perceives that a clinical culture can be improved and he or she pioneers new attitudes and approaches in the field.

However, if a student feels out of place among practitioners in the field despite efforts to adapt, it may portend a challenging interpersonal dynamic. It may benefit the student to look at other fields of training where there may be a more natural, collegial fit with other practitioners.

In addition to needing to work closely with colleagues, a practitioner will need to work closely with the patients he or she serves. Students should consider what kind of patient and patient service is most compatible with their personality. As an example, if a student enjoys short-term relationships, then emergency medicine or anesthesiology may make a good fit. If interested in long-term relationships and longitudinal care, then family or internal medicine might be more appropriate. If a student has a natural skill working with children and parents, pediatrics would seem to be a good choice. If a student does not enjoy working with patients directly but is interested in making indirect contributions to patient care, then radiology or pathology might be most compatible with the student's personal goals.

5. Other Considerations

The four factors described above that influence a student's career choice are not comprehensive. Other considerations may be paramount for some students. For example, geography can be important. A student who has a strong preference for living in a rural setting may not want to train in neurosurgery because nearly all jobs are based in urban areas. The duration of training also is extremely important to some students. A student interested in basic-science research may be reluctant to train in a field that requires long and intense surgical training because such training may create a large gap before allowing a return to research.

Thus, while aptitude, interest, values and work-life balance, and people are important to assess, there may be other factors of equal or greater importance that need to be included in a student's career decision making.

GATHERING DATA BEFORE CHOOSING A MEDICAL CAREER

Clinical clerkships are perhaps the most widely used immersive experiences to test a field for potential fit for postgraduate training and a future career. Most residency programs encourage at least two exposures—a core and an advanced clerkship (or subinternship) in the field—before submitting a residency application.

In addition, most medical schools support diverse activities that allow students to actively explore their career interests early in medical school. These activities include:

Student-faculty interest groups. Most medical schools have established groups or clubs that foster mentorship and information exchange among students, house staff, and attending physicians in different fields of practice. At Stanford, we have approximately 15 student-initiated interest groups, spanning from internal medicine to otolaryngology/head and neck surgery, that meet approximately quarterly and allow such a dialogue. Many faculty members are keen to be "adopted" by students as role models and they enjoy mentoring students interested in exploring their fields.

Early elective coursework. Elective coursework is often available to pre-clerkship students, allowing an early exposure to a variety of training fields. These electives can be classroom-based or immersive. At Stanford, for instance, we offer pre-clerkship students a course in vascular surgery that includes a didactic component and simulation exercises to teach students how to suture and create vascular anastomoses.

Shadowing experiences. Early shadowing experiences provide an opportunity for pre-clerkship students to observe the day-to-day workings of a clinician.

Most clinical shadowing is limited to two to four hours at a time. As implied by the name, shadowing has inherent limitations because students are peripheral to patient care (as opposed to clerkships, where they are actively managing patients). Nevertheless, students often find these experiences useful as a first introduction to the field. Because of the relatively short exposure, students can often complete several shadowing experiences during the 12–24 months of pre-clerkship training.

Friends, academic advisors, books. These are additional resources that can inform a student about the potential positive and negative attributes of fields of training. Peer-to-peer counseling and advice from friends, faculty, and academic advisors can be useful. Widely used resources include:

- *Getting into a Residency* by K.V. Iserson (2013, Galen Press, Tucson, AZ);
- *The Ultimate Guide to Choosing a Medical Specialty* by B. Freeman. (2013, McGraw Hill, New York, NY);
- *How to Choose a Medical Specialty* by A.D. Taylor (2013, Publish Green, Minneapolis, MN); and
- *On Becoming a Doctor* by T. Heller (2009, Sourcebooks, Naperville, IL).

This is not a comprehensive list, and it seems that "how to" books that provide advice on how to apply for residency and succeed in the residency match, are plentiful.

A PRACTICAL ALGORITHM FOR CHOOSING A MEDICAL CAREER

Armed with information gathered from pre-clerkship experiences and the other tools described above, medical students enter clinical clerkship training, which is often the immersive testing ground to explore potential fields for clinical training in detail. At Stanford, we have used a simple and practical algorithm (Figure 2-1) to provide a framework that defines decision points for making a career choice.

The assumption of the algorithm is that each medical student will complete the requirements for the MD degree. The algorithm has several decision points, shown in the figure by boxes A, B, and C.

Decision point A involves the student deciding whether he or she will be a practicing physician or use the MD degree for an alternative career. At Stanford, about 2–5% of students each year elect to use the MD degree to pursue alternative careers in areas such as biomedical research, biotechnology, healthcare consulting, public health, health policy, medical journalism, and medical education.

Although this pathway does not require residency training, physicians who do not complete postgraduate training are not eligible for licensure, which often creates a "ceiling" effect as to how far MD graduates can progress in their chosen

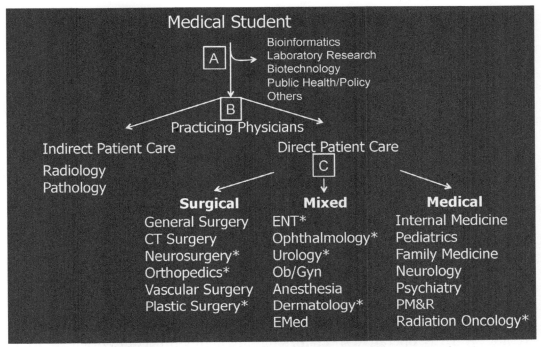

Figure 2-1. A Career in Medicine Algorithm. (*Extremely competitive for the residency match)

field. We usually encourage students to complete at least one year of postgraduate training so they can become licensed, even if they plan to pursue one of these alternative fields.

Decision point B involves the student deciding whether he or she will be involved in indirect or direct patient care. Two fields, radiology and pathology, are shown in this diagram as fields where physicians provide indirect patient care; that is, they provide valuable information (imaging and clinical/pathological diagnostics, respectively) that are used by other physicians in the care of patients. Interventional radiologists are an exception because they do have direct patient contact and responsibilities.

Decision point C, under direct patient care, is the destination of the majority of medical students. In our advising system, we have found it useful to ask students to reflect on whether they have a predominantly surgical or medical orientation to patient care. The medical–surgical dichotomy is useful in guiding the decision toward possible fields of training.

A surgical orientation (left side under decision point C) is evident in students who are keen to "fix" things, to have more immediate results, to use surgical techniques to repair or replace organs and tissues. Surgically oriented students enjoy the operating room, almost to a fault. They find surgeries exciting and cannot envision a future career devoid of significant time in the operating room. Surgically oriented students are willing to make personal and time sacrifices to earn the opportunity for operative training and experience.

Students with a medical orientation (right side under decision point C) are less interested in surgery and immediate outcomes. They are highly analytical and more willing to engage in long-term treatment and care. The length of training is usually shorter than surgical training, although fellowship training, for instance in internal medicine and pediatrics, can extend total postgraduate training time to 5–7 years.

Some fields of clinical training (center, "mixed" column under decision point C) offer opportunities for surgery or are highly procedural, but also include medical training. For example, obstetrics and gynecology requires significant training in the operating and delivery rooms; once in practice, however, obstetrics/gynecology practitioners can decide to be mostly office-based and not spend significant time in surgery. Specialties such as emergency medicine, anesthesiology, and dermatology are not primarily operative specialties but are highly procedure-oriented; thus, they provide satisfaction to students with both medical and surgical orientations.

The areas of training shown with an asterisk (*) are extremely competitive for the residency match. For students applying in these asterisked fields, completing research within the field of training often is necessary to compete for a training position. In addition to published scholarship, students competing for training in these fields need to be a "triple threat": strong in clinical performance, strong in professionalism, and strong in discipline-specific scholarship.

SUMMARY

Choosing a field for postgraduate training is the most important career decision a student makes in medical school. The advice we give to students choosing a field for training is this: first and most importantly, pick a discipline that you are passionate about; second, make sure you have sufficient aptitude for and interest in the discipline; third, ensure that training and clinical practice are compatible with your values and desire for work-life balance; and fourth, identify a field of training where you resonate with the people in the field—both the practitioners you work with and the patients you serve. Although a perfect career match can be elusive, most students find their niche in medicine using these principles.

The author did not receive any financial support in creating this review. There are no conflicts of interest.

CHAPTER 3

Landing Your First Job: The Essentials

Keith Borglum, CHBC CBB

THOUSANDS OF PHYSICIANS FACE career opportunities every year. Many are graduating residents and fellows, but career change can present itself anywhere along a physician's life. All physicians face three career options: get a job, buy a practice, or start a practice.

Despite the best-laid career plans, sometimes things don't work out and a career change becomes necessary or desirable for a physician. Some are early-career physicians who decide they made a mistake in choosing an employer or in choosing a location in which to practice. Some found that the position they were planning to take evaporated. Some planned from the beginning to work for someone else, getting comfortable with their clinical and business skills before they went out on their own.

Some are mid-career doctors whose groups break up or whose groups are acquired by a bigger group with whom they find they disagree. Some divorce from their marital/practice partners, have a mid-life crisis, or relocate to follow a new spouse. Others leave their current situations to form new groups or concierge practices. Even senior physicians sometimes find themselves in a situation where going independent is the "lesser of the evils" prior to retiring in a few years.

The data remain anecdotal as yet, but practice management consultants are seeing increasing numbers of physicians who have been in practice 3–20 years coming to them for practice restarts, including practice purchases, jobs, and startups from scratch. It's a trickle now, but it could become a flood given demographic and economic trajectories in the United States. A few banks even have divisions specializing in funding physician and dental startups, acquisitions, expansions, and mergers.

Payors are unhappy with the higher costs of hospital-employed physicians. If legislation eliminates the higher fees hospitals can charge for their employed physicians due to Point of Service codes, it will cause a flood of physician restarts or retirements when the hospitals fold, fire all the physicians, or cut the physicians' pay so much they leave. It happened in the 1990s after the last binge of hospitals acquired then released physician practices, and it could happen again.

New medical school grads probably have the hardest time finding their way. They are facing the most significant change in circumstances since they left for college. They are leaving a clear path within a structured institutional environment and venturing into the unknown.

According to one survey, "92% of residents indicated they would prefer to be employed with a salary than an independent practice guarantee or loan. 36% indicated they would prefer to be employed by a hospital rather than any other job option. Only 2% of residents indicated they would prefer a solo setting as their first practice. 48% said they are unprepared to handle the business side of medicine. Residents identified 'geographic location,' 'personal time,' and 'lifestyle' as their most important considerations when evaluating a medical practice opportunity. Only 7% would prefer to practice in communities of 50,000 or less. 46% said they have been contacted by recruiters 100 or more times during the course of their training. 25% of residents indicated that, were they to begin their education again, they would choose a field other than medicine."[1]

If this is your first practice, or if you are coming out of residency or fellowship, you will be experiencing the biggest personal economic change of your life as well. Plan your budget to live on no more than 75% of your after-tax income. It's how much money you keep—not how much you make—that counts!

FIND YOUR PLACE AND YOUR NICHE

As faculty for several medical associations and residencies, I'm often asked "Where should I open my practice?"—as if there is some enchanted city that will guarantee success. The best place to start a practice is *where you want to spend the rest of your life outside of practice*. In other words, when you leave the office at the end of your long day, close the door and turn around to face the world, be where you want to live, irrespective of economics and income. Most exam rooms and hallways look the same everywhere.

There are few places in the United States that can't use another physician in your specialty, or where your practice would not be reasonably successful. Why not have a practice where you want to live, or live where you would otherwise want to vacation? Even those locations that might be considered heavily over-doctored will probably have a niche community within a two-hour drive.

Recognize that the more over-saturated the market, the fewer the income opportunities. A saying in Southern California is "you can practice at the beach and only afford to live inland, or you can practice inland and be able to afford to live at the beach." The best income opportunities are often more than an hour from a coast, ski resort, resort community, or urban center.

Aside from some urban super-specialists, most of my clients who net over $1 million per year are in secondary and tertiary markets. A primary market has 5 million or more people. A secondary market has 2 million to 5 million people. A tertiary market is under 2 million people. From the conservative viewpoint, primary markets could be as narrowly defined as the top five metro areas in the United States: Los Angeles, San Francisco, New York, Chicago, and Washington, DC. Orange County, considered by many to be a primary market, has Yorba Linda and Santa Ana, which are arguably not primary areas. Similarly, Los Angeles has Palmdale and Lancaster, which have much more tertiary-market characteristics. All U.S. states not included in major metro areas and secondary markets are tertiary.

Studies suggest that money only buys happiness up to around $50,000 per year— enough to cover basic necessities—then has no further direct impact on personal happiness, so look beyond the potential practice income in selecting a location. If otherwise in doubt, be near family. I regularly broker practices to buyers who relocate to be near aging and ailing parents.

An ophthalmologist client who struggled financially in a California resort area moved to a smaller town in the Midwest to be near his aging parents and imme-diately quadrupled his income. Now he has more time off and money to relax and visit in his old resort community than when he lived there full time. Another physician had a girlfriend in Rio de Janeiro, Brazil. He and three other physicians split a three-person practice in a not-so-great city; they each worked three months on and one month off in a year-round rotation, each earning enough income to be happy—especially during their month-long vacations.

Many other physicians have a long weekend or a long week off (a week off plus two weekend on each side) every six weeks and still work 48 weeks per year. No matter where you settle down, book your vacations in advance, and get out of town!

If you want more tangible evidence to support your choice of locale, do your own research rather than buying a demographic survey. Have someone pose as the son or daughter of an aging parent who needs a simple routine evaluation in your specialty, and call around to the majority of medical offices in that specialty to find out the wait time for a new appointment. Most patients like to be seen within a week or two of calling for an appointment. If the response is, "What time today would you like to come in?" it will be a tough locale for a new physician. For every two weeks of wait, there is room for another physician. If the only physi-cian in town has a two-week wait, then adding a physician would result in two physicians each having a one-week wait time. If three physicians in a community each have a four-week wait time, then there is room for six or more physicians and you will need to do virtually no marketing other than sending an announcement to the potential referrers and competitors in the community; your wait-list will probably equal theirs within months.

An ongoing patient waiting list of more than one day means you still have a full practice; if you always have a full day of appointments, you are full. One plastic surgeon asked me to help him with marketing because his wait-list for face-lifts had dropped from six months to four months. I recommended that he double his fees, then double them again after another six months. He still has a months-long wait list, but now understands "market balance" and will be able to retire years earlier if he so chooses. When patients question his high price, he tells them he'd be happy to refer them to some good "half-price" surgeons if they can't afford him. Most choose to wait.

Another plastic surgeon in the same city only does cosmetic rhinoplasties because that's what he likes to do. His niche is the "new nose in 30 days for $99/month," with most of his clients being middle- and lower-middle class working persons. He is in the same geographic market as the prior surgeon, but with an entirely different population. Both have full and successful practices. So, find your niche wherever you want to practice.

GET A JOB

It's a great time for new physicians to find a job. There have never been so many jobs available with so many types of large institutional employers—private, corporate, academic, or military—and it's much easier to take a job with a big institution when you are coming straight out of the structured education system because you haven't had a taste of the control and satisfaction (despite the hassles) of private practice.

According to the American Association of Medical Colleges, "By 2020 the nation will face a shortage of 45,000 PCPs and 46,000 specialists and surgeons. Unless Congress lifts the 16-year-old cap on federal support for residency training, we will still face a shortfall of physicians across dozens of specialties"[2]

This shortage is due in part to the Patient Protection and Affordable Care Act (PPACA), which "re-corporatized" healthcare after the semi-failure of the HMO and Physician Practice Management Company (PPMC) movements. "All a person has to do is pick up a newspaper to see the biggest challenge facing the health care provider sector: implementation of the Affordable Care Act and all of its legislative- and market-driven implications."[3]

This concern is further supported by the large health reform consultancies like McKinsey & Co., with statements to physician-employers and payors such as this: "Because the widespread use of outcomes-based payments will significantly increase performance pressure on providers, . . . if providers are to bear financial accountability for the cost and quality of the care they deliver, they must face a meaningful level of downside risk," and, according to the McKinsey & Co. report, "50% or more of each provider's revenue should be outcomes-based and hence, at risk."[4]

A March 2013 report by the Society of Actuaries—the nation's leading group of financial risk analysts—predicts that "PPACA claims costs filed by individual policy holders (i.e., those without employer-provided plans) could rise by as much as 32% nationally and 62% in California by 2017, increasing prices for patients and thwarting health reform. Even some former administration advisers say a new round of cost-curbing legislation will be needed."[5] This will likely include further cuts to physician compensation.

Still, taking a job with a large employer is a pretty safe bet. It comes with a regular paycheck, maybe a signing bonus, maybe productivity and quality bonuses, and a staff and systems in place—all you have to do is fit in. According to the American Academy of Family Physicians surveys, the desire to attain a certain degree of income security and reduce the pressure of administration burdens is driving physicians to seek the security of practicing medicine as employees rather than as business owners.[6] When a large organization fails, it usually gets swallowed up by a larger organization and often all that changes is the employer's name on the physician's paycheck, but sometimes also the size of that paycheck.

According to a 2013 article in *Forbes*, a cut in pay for hospital-employed physicians is likely.

> "For Obamacare to succeed, American doctors need to earn less money. At present issue are the rates paid to doctors working as part of hospital-owned clinics versus physicians working in their own, independent offices. Right now, when a doctor works as part of hospital-owned practice and bills Medicare, the hospital/employer is paid more money than what the physician would receive for providing the same services in his or her own independent medical office. That's because of an arbitrage between Medicare's inpatient (Part A) and outpatient (Part B) billing schemes. In order to take advantage of these differentials, hospitals have gone on a buying binge in recent years, purchasing doctor practices. One of their aims was to bring the physicians' services (and the procedures that doctors perform) under the "Part A" reimbursement scheme, where they can bill at higher

rates for the same services. In fact, for hospitals, outpatient services are among their highest profit centers (typically, along with neonatal intensive care units and spine surgery). For doctors, coming under the "Part A" billing scheme was a way to offset their declining incomes, and lock in long-term employment agreements with hospitals. It was also a way to foist the rising cost of running their outpatient medical practices onto the hospitals (and stem reductions in their real income as they saw their reimbursement levels held flat, or slightly decline, while their practice costs rose.) But the Medicare Payment Advisory Commission (MedPAC) said that reimbursement rates should be made "site neutral." In other words, the price arbitrage between Medicare's outpatient and inpatient billing schemes should be ended. To accommodate these costly mandates, and still keep the health plans cheap, insurers need to control what providers do, and limit what they're paid. By one example, the Medicare Payment Advisory Commission proposed to cut what Medicare pays specialists and then freezing these lower rates for years. Under that plan, everyone except primary-care doctors would see payments for their services cut by 5.9% a year for 3 years (totaling a 16.7% cut in income), followed by a 7-year freeze at the reduced levels. Primary-care providers would have their reimbursement rates frozen at today's pay levels for the whole decade."[7]

Certainly no Medicare provision of reform has generated more interest than the Medicare Shared Savings Program (MSSP) for ACOs or accountable care organizations. According to CMS, an ACO is "a new kind of provider organization whose members (physicians, hospitals and most related services) share responsibility for care quality, financial risk, and a common goal to improve health care delivery and the overall health status for a given population of Medicare beneficiaries." In short, ACOs are a re-invention of the health maintenance organizations, (HMOs), with several new twists.

A newer twist is the creation and expansion of a larger mix of organizations referred to as Emerging Healthcare Organizations (EHOs). One of these new EHO/ACO models is driven by more and more insurance company purchases of medical practices. "In southern California, where some of the purchases have occurred, the insurers are jockeying with hospitals and physician groups for bargaining power," notes Wells Shoemaker, M.D., medical director of the California Association of Physician Groups. "As consolidation of providers and insurers grows," he says, "hospitals, physician groups and health plans all are increasingly nervous about being outmaneuvered. WellPoint acquired a 26-office physician organization in southern California. Optum bought Orange County's Monarch HealthCare and two smaller IPAs. Optum also controls medical management companies in Arizona and Texas, and sister company UnitedHealthcare acquired a multispecialty group in Nevada as part of its purchase of Sierra Health & Life, a smaller insurance firm. Humana purchased Concentra, which provides occupational care and other medical services at more than 300 stand-alone clinics and 240 work-site facilities. United and Optum are buying also, and CIGNA has a private-label plan with Houston's Kelsey-Seybold Clinic. Back in California, where it all started, Blue Shield of California has been running an ACO pilot on behalf of CalPERS, the state retirement system. Its partners in this Sacramento-based endeavor are Hill Physicians—a big IPA—and Dignity Health (formerly the Catholic Healthcare West hospital chain). Blue Shield is now moving ahead with 20 similar ACOs."[8]

In those markets there are fewer and fewer opportunities for independent medical practices and physicians. In 2013 in California, Blue Cross cut half the physicians, and Health Net reduced 65% of its primary care physicians. Medicare itself is supporting those insurance/ACO models—and competing with independent physicians—by providing lists of all Medicare patients to the ACOs—referencing their physicians' names—with which to convert patients from their current physicians.

Not long ago, most insurers wanted a broad panel of doctors and hospitals to contact as participating providers in a health plan, but insurance companies are now creating insurance products with narrow panels. "These chains of providers—also called Narrow Networks or high-value quality or select networks—judge practices by cost and quality metrics and eliminate some practices from their list of participating providers. Narrow network plans have grown in popularity particularly due to PPACA because of their cheaper premiums. About 70% of plans sold on the exchanges in 2014 featured a narrow network. In California, customers filed a class-action lawsuit against Anthem, Blue Shield of California and Cigna for allegedly deceiving customers about which hospitals and doctors participated in their limited networks. Plaintiffs called the plans a "bait and switch."[9]

Narrow networks can leave a lot of independent doctors without historic insurance contracts, like with Blue Cross, Blue Shield, Aetna, etc. Aetna has announced ACO contracts with two provider organizations, and it is in discussions with 130 health care systems and physician groups. Aetna's preferred strategy is to turn ACOs into narrow networks that it can sell under their own names as private-label plans. Aetna isn't the only insurer promoting narrow networks based on ACOs. "The designation is strictly based on claims/cost data; not necessarily on quality," says Marcia Brauchler, MPH, CPC-I, CPHQ, president, Physicians' Ally, Inc., Littleton, Colo. "If you're a provider and you're participating in these managed care plans, you better know if you're being evaluated, and on which metrics. Payer data is incomplete; 'quality' is an amorphous, nebulous word that can be defined by anyone and everyone a million-plus different ways; and providers, as always, are reactive rather than proactive." "The only way to talk 'quality' on even somewhat equitable terms is to have your own data to back your position. The vast majority of providers have no idea how to get clear, well-defined data from their own systems to have the conversation, and the complexity is only increasing"[10]

Large corporations are beginning to acquire medical groups to build ACOs. For example DaVita, the country's largest renal dialysis company, bought Healthcare Partners. "DaVita's acquisition of HealthCare Partners, which has 700 employed physicians and a network of 8,300 independent doctors, gives it a stronger foothold in accountable care organizations, which are a significant part of the Patient Protection and Affordable Care Act. HealthCare Partners is one of the Pioneer Accountable Care Organizations named by the Centers for Medicare & Medicaid Services. It also participates in the ACO pilot project for people covered by Anthem Blue CrossDaVita's Paladina Health subsidiary earlier acquired ModernMed, which had 30 clinics in 12 states providing primary care to patients paying a membership fee."[11]

Independent Physician Associations (IPAs) are also ACO contenders. According to one IPA, "We see moving from IPA to ACO status as perhaps the most important opportunity ever for physicians to retain their independence and ownership, and to benefit financially from providing high quality, efficient care. Our IPA is primary care-based, and we're committed to the idea of the Patient-Centered Medical Home (PCMH). But we're extending the PCMH concept to include outpatient specialty care for most chronic illnesses, and we think we can save patients and payers like Medicare a lot of money through close coordination of care. You could say we're creating an ACO that is a PCMH neighborhood."[12] Unfortunately, few have the financial resources to do so, and an IPA failure hurts independent physicians in that market.

Retail clinics are expanding competition. As of September 2014, CVS Pharmacy is the largest provider of retail-based health clinics in the US, with plans to grow to 1,500 clinics by 2017.[13] Walmart has announced a challenge with its intent to "become the nation's largest primary care provider," placing over 2,500 Solo-Health unstaffed kiosks, in addition to its 140 clinics. Target trails with 80 clinics, and is a takeover target.

"There is a trend in general by retailers and health insurers to provide 'fluff' to consumers in the guise of real medical information as an advertising delivery device," says the group Consumer Watchdog. CVS/Caremark, Walgreen's, Kroger, Target and others have recently reinvigorated efforts to open in-store medical clinics. Walmart was the nation's leader in opening such clinics, but has dropped to third place, well behind industry leader CVS Caremark's nearly 550 Minute

Clinics and Walgreen's 355 Take Care clinics, according to data tracked by Tom Charland, CEO of Merchant Medicine, a Minnesota-based research and consulting firm. About 1,500 store-based clinics are open nationwide, he says. They have different business models. Walmart leases space to independent vendors in 90 clinics, but is moving to the CVS model, wherein CVS owns and staffs its Minute Clinics. Walmart–the largest employer in the US–charges $40/visit to the public, and $4/visit to employees and dependents, also accepting Medicare. While a few centers operated by retailers have doctors on site, most hire nurse practitioners or physician assistants to provide the care. "This is an industry where people haven't figured out how to make money," he says.[14]

Blue Cross in late 2015 made tele-medicine a member benefit at $49 per online visit, so jobs in telemedicine should significantly increase.

DOING YOUR HOMEWORK

Most new physicians join a practice without first giving it a thorough "history and physical." By asking pertinent questions up front—before you join the practice—you can save yourself a lot of aggravation. First, it will help you avoid joining a practice that isn't the right fit for you. Second, knowing your rights in the practice ahead of time will help avoid legal problems in the future. Here are some suggestions:

- Visit a practice for at least a full day, or up to a week, giving people a chance to show their true selves rather than their "interview personalities."
- Call the medical director or chief of staff of the hospital where the group has privileges and ask questions. If the feedback is lukewarm or guarded, you'll be able to read between the lines.
- Do some research in the community. Does the practice have a bad reputation or bad publicity in the community for any apparent reason?
- If it's a small or independent group employer, have an accountant or independent medical practice management consultant perform a Practice Survey and tell you if it is a good opportunity, if the accounting is questionable, or if the practice is going broke. A consultant can uncover some hidden problems that an inexperienced person might miss.
- Consider whether the incentives are reasonable or so unrealistic that no newcomer could expect to reach them.
- Is achievement of your incentive based on the competence of their billing office?
- Is there an income guarantee? How long? Guaranteed by whom? Then what?
- Check out the turnover history of other associates in the practice to see if there's a revolving door situation.

- Don't just accept the word of management that you will be accepted into the managed care plans; get it in writing from the plans themselves.
- Get any ownership terms and price in writing in advance, including the buy-in formula. Are any senior owners planning to retire and expect to be bought-out by the other shareholders? If so, at what price? Is that why they are bringing you in?
- What kind of plan is available if things don't work out? If you decide after a few months that the practice is not for you, can you walk away without major obligations?
- Who is in charge of the practice? Remember, staff really run the practice and often know more than the doctors about what is going on.
- What is the frequency of staff meetings? If staff members don't get together at least once a month, expect some communication problems and unresolved issues.
- Do employees have clear job descriptions?
- Do the doctors handle the employees professionally, or are they at risk for a lawsuit? Does any doctor refer to staff members as sweetheart or darling—or vice versa?
- If you're considering joining a small group with nepotistic tendencies, what happens if you have a problem with a staff-family member?
- Check the schedule & EMR, computer, lab transmittals, hospital relationships, and everything else to see if the practice is organized and up-to-date. Is EMR implementation or conversion planned? If so, you might want to wait until it's completed.
- If the practice has an employment and governance document that spells everything out on paper, wonderful! It's more likely that they have the bare bones of an employment or partnership contract, 95% legalese, and often out of date. Work with your lawyer or a practice management consultant to list everything on the document that could affect you in the future. Then run the paperwork by a medical practice specialist attorney. I've seen five-year contracts wherein the employer can cancel with 90 days' notice—and they have. Go to the Superior Court and look for history of litigation against the group or have your attorney do it.
- Is your personal space an office, a cubbyhole, or a spot referred to as "we'll work that out"? Some physicians function very well sharing a desk in a noisy environment—others need those four walls and a door to get through the day.
- Patient distribution refers to how patients are divided up in the practice. Does the new physician get all the troublesome patients the other doctors don't want to see?
- Who's going to show you the ropes? Or are you just expected to absorb things through osmosis?

Get everything in writing or risk future problems!

Summary

ACOs, EHOs, IPAs, hospitals, drug stores, retailers, insurance plans, corporate partners, narrow networks—which will be the best and safest employer? It's anyone's guess, but in real life, Goliath usually beats David.

With regard to negotiations, typically, there's no sense trying—it's a corporate environment, so take it or leave it. Don't waste time trying to change it unless the position is with a smaller, non-institutional group.

To find a job in your specialty, it's as easy as Googling it—you will get lots of hits. To find out market rates of compensation, buy the MGMA's *Physician Compensation and Production Report,* which is the same report that most employers use to set pay scales.

BUY A JOB

You can "buy a job" by buying a practice. Buying a practice at the "right price" may prove to be the best investment you will ever make in your professional life, bar none. In general, 60%–75% annual rates of return are common (think of it as getting a 65% interest rate on savings).

Given the national shortage and mal-distribution of physicians, it has never been easier to buy the practice of a successful retiring physician at an attractive price. Because so many physicians are taking employment with large organizations, retiring physicians with excellent practices in great locations often must simply close their practices without selling them because associates and buyers (even at zero price) aren't interested.

As a professional practice broker for 30 years, I discovered that most candidates willing to buy practices during the past decade are foreign medical graduates—or the offspring or families of such—from cultures where independence and business pride-of-ownership attitudes are still strong. My business broker colleagues outside of medicine report the same thing in their fields of specialization, so it appears to be at least partly a cultural issue, not medical-specific.

Other excellent practice-purchase candidates are physicians who have been employed by a group for 3–5 years, are comfortable with their clinical skills, and now hate their jobs because of the lack of control they have.

Sometimes, buying a practice is the only way into a particular community, since all of the local insurance plans and networks are closed to new physicians. Some plans allow a new physician in as "an associate" of a currently enrolled member, as long as the new physician was an associate for six months prior to taking over. Have your attorney read the contracts to investigate this issue. Sometimes contracts may indicate something like, "If 50% or more of shares are sold, the contract can be terminated by the plan."

When buying a practice, you have the advantage of quicker cash flow, fewer marketing expenses, and less work to assemble the components of the practice. On the other hand, a purchased practice probably is not exactly what you would want if you had built it from scratch; you may need to make some modification or relocate after a year or two, or at lease expiration.

Physicians who are about to start their own practice often wonder whether it is more or less expensive to start a practice from scratch versus buying one. The answer depends on the price and details of an available practice. It is less expensive to buy a practice at or below fair market value (FMV) than to start your own; however it is less expensive to start a practice from scratch than to over-pay for a purchase. With employment compensation, both scenarios balance each other out financially, which is what keeps FMV "fair."

Don't confuse value with price. Value is determined by a qualified, impartial, and disinterested person based on a set of assumptions—for example, whether Medicare reimbursement will go up or down in the future; price is negotiated. Valuation is a product of both professional judgment and professional opinion. Successful negotiation between two individuals, each with his or her own perceived value of a practice, results in a price.

In a practice transaction, a buyer and a seller, each with a personal motivation, negotiate price under specific circumstances. To estimate value, a professional appraiser makes assumptions regarding standards of value and premises of value, both terms of which have much published and many court cases about them have been decided. The standard of value applied to a particular appraisal will be determined by the requirements of law, such as in a divorce or estate proceeding, or by the preferences of the client with the agreement of the appraiser.

A premise of value differs from a standard of value in that it identifies the assumption upon which the appraisal reasoning proceeds, such as a fair market value under the premise of a going concern or under the premise of forced liquidation.

The optimal premise for viewing a particular set of assets depends on the purpose of an appraisal. If, for example, a prospective buyer wished to know the value of a target doctor's practice for purposes of buying and continuing the practice, he or she would be best served by an appraisal on the premise of going concern. A lender who wanted to test the adequacy of the same practice as collateral for a loan typically would be safer with an appraisal on a premise of liquidation.

In most cases, both the buyer and seller of a medical practice are interested in the fair market value under the premise of a going concern, which means the value of the practice if operated in a normal and customary basis. The financial value of a practice primarily boils down to two standards:

1. Fair market value with a return on investment and a return of investment, through earnings above what you could earn in similar employment with a group; and
2. Strategic/Investment value wherein you are willing to pay more than fair market value because you want to be in that particular locale, there are no jobs available, and you can't or don't want to start one there from scratch.

Practice Value

Practice value has two parts: tangible assets and intangible assets (often described as "goodwill" value). Tangible assets like exam tables, leasehold improvements, instrumentation, EMR, and furnishings are relatively easy to value. "Intangible" or "goodwill" is what is difficult to value, and usually requires a healthcare appraisal expert.

People often confuse the concept of "sociological goodwill" with "financial goodwill." Sellers wonder why their practice has little-or-no dollar value of goodwill when they have an excellent reputation, have a large patient following, and have poured years of blood, sweat, and tears into their businesses. The answer is that if the sociological goodwill doesn't demonstrate itself in dollars (i.e., dividends as well-described by IRS Revenue Ruling 59–60—income above compensation for labor), then the sociological goodwill has no measure or value when measured in dollars.

According to valuation principals, an intangible asset needs certain characteristics to have value. It should generate some measurable amount of economic income to its owner. This economic benefit could be in the form of an income increment or a cost decrement. An example of a source of income increment is a sole owner of a practice that profitably employs midlevel providers and ancillary services like imaging or lab, wherein there is net income above what they would earn in just self-employment. When you are solo, and your earnings are dependent on your own ICD/CPT billings, you are only being paid compensation for your labor, without compensation for ownership.

The opportunity for a buyer to take the existing practice and build upon it has no goodwill value either because that the result of the buyer's efforts (above those demonstrated by the seller) and belongs to the buyer, not to the seller.

This brings up the issue of buying an entity, like a corporation or LLC, or buying the assets. By far, most small practice sales are "asset sales" wherein the buyer acquires the practice without the "corporate shell." The corporate shell, along with its malpractice and corporate liabilities like labor disputes, remains with the seller. On the other hand, most buy-ins to groups are for shares in the entity. Sometimes the sale of the entire practice does include the entity so that the buyer can keep any preferential contracts of the entity (like insurance plan contracts), but the buyer then inherits liabilities that likely should be insured against, and perhaps unresolved tax liabilities. Sole proprietorships never sell the entity because there is no entity to sell.

The rules are arcane and often illogical, and even Medicare has rules on the topic. Therefore, use a specialist attorney who has done dozens, hundreds or thousands of transactions. The specialist attorney will keep you out of trouble. You can find them by referral through your national medical association or specialty associations like the National Society of Certified Healthcare Business Consultants (NSCHBC.org), the Medical Group Management Association (MGMA.com), or the American Health Lawyers Association (HealthLawyers.org).

Even if you are using a practice broker with a specialty in healthcare to buy a practice, use an attorney also. Most states require that you need a state license to cut hair, but they don't require that practice brokers be licensed or trained. In states that do license business brokers, most states only allow the business brokers to use fill-in-the-blank forms that are fine for selling a restaurant or laundromat, but not for selling a medical practice that requires state and federal compliance. A broker who is not using the state-approved form is considered performing the unlicensed practice of law, which can cause legal issues for you if you use an unlicensed "broker" no matter the fancy name they might call themselves like "transaction consultant."

You wouldn't use unlicensed doctors, so don't use unlicensed, uncertified brokers. You can find legitimate brokers listed at the National Association of Certified Healthcare Business Consultants (NSCHBC.org) or by a search on the Internet for "medical practice broker."

Here are some guidelines when considering a broker:

- Beware of websites or companies that don't list the broker's personal name or license number prominently (required by law in many states).
- Beware of new brokers who bought the practice of an experienced broker and now claim the company's experience-in-years as their own. Also beware of brokers who are just renting an agent "seat" from a broker. Ask the broker or agent how many medical practices they personally have brokered.

- Beware of companies with no licenses, certifications, or medical-practice credentials posted.
- Beware of companies that serve dentists for the part, as that is its own specialty market.
- Beware of companies with no specific content on their websites, just platitudes.
- Beware of companies whose "broker" is an "affiliate" or "partner" and is just splitting fees splitting with the advertiser.
- Beware of companies that say "they will do all the paperwork," especially if they are a "dual representation firm" or "dual agency," ostensibly serving both parties to the transaction.
- Beware of brokerages wherein the office photos are all the same photo or "coming soon." Most practice sellers should remain confidential and photos could violate confidentiality.
- Beware of brokerages whose information is full of mis-spellings and poor grammar—like this: "Multi-specialty Medi-Care surgery center—Los Angeles, CA. This ASC is of a kind in the county."
- Beware of criminal history. Do an Internet search about the individual broker who will be working with you. You might find information like this: "was sentenced to three years in prison for racketeering and received a five-year suspended sentence for obstruction of justice. He also was fined $45,000. He agreed to forfeit $1 million to the government as part of his plea agreement."

Use a non-specialist attorney at your own peril. I was a leasehold-value expert in a litigation wherein the physician sublet a satellite office part-time from a chiropractor, without having his medical attorney review the lease and protections. The chiropractor was sued for malpractice. Because the physician's name was on the door, he also was sued. Prior to deposing the physician, the plaintiff's attorney notified HIPAA that there might be a privacy violation (without any basis in fact). The plaintiff's attorney also notified the state medical board that there might be a sublet fee-splitting violation due to off-market rent rates to encourage referral (without any basis in fact). Both HIPAA and the medical board were then required by law to investigate.

When the attorney deposed the physician in the chiropractic malpractice case, he asked two questions: "Isn't it true, doctor, that in addition to being 'involved' (without any basis in fact) during the injury that occurred to my client, you are also being investigated by the Federal Government for violation of patient privacy—true or false?" And "Isn't it true, doctor, that in addition to being involved during the injury that occurred to my client, and also being investigated by the Federal Government for violation of patient privacy, you are also being investigated by your own state medical board for possible felony fee splitting—true or false?" This is why you pay an attorney a "relatively" small amount in advance, rather than a large amount later. This innocent physician paid $70,000 in fees and settlement costs.

Buying a practice is harder than just taking a job, but possibly more satisfying. On the other hand it is usually significantly easier than starting from scratch. It might be worthwhile to a physician starting a practice to first ask the older doctors in the community if they might be interested in selling their practice. Otherwise, most practices for sale can be found on just a handful of websites including BizBuySell. com, MergerNetwork.com, BizQuest.com, and perhaps your own specialty's website. And in all cases, use an experienced specialist attorney to represent you.

CREATE A JOB

Starting a practice from scratch is harder than taking a job or buying a practice, but hundreds of thousands of doctors have done it successfully. You can do it too. In fewer than 10 hours, a healthcare practice management consultant can educate you on how to open and run a practice, and after another 100 hours of physician effort over a few months, you can be seeing your first patient.

As a variation of starting a practice, you might consider forming or joining a partnership of professional independent practices. When done correctly, this strategy can give the new doctor a lot of independence in practice, some of the benefits of being in a group, and the ability to share in some ancillary services that might otherwise be prohibited by Stark or Medicare fee-splitting laws like labs and imaging. Other benefits can include separate retirement plans, central-ized administration, shared and more-expert billing, shared electronic healthcare records, fewer staffing hassles, etc.

If considering joining an established organization, you should critically examine the established entity, its fee structure, governance, and get review by a specialist-attorney to make sure it is set up correctly. Surprisingly, some are not set up correctly; which can lead to a lot of trouble later if there is a malpractice or professional-liability incident. If starting a practice from scratch, the extra expense of a specialist-attorney is required, but the lawyers who specialize in this usually have some "canned" structures you can cost-effectively adopt.

Be cautious about hospital income guarantees (forgivable loans) if offered. The devil is in the details; terms differ widely and may or may not be a good deal for your individual situation. Be aware that the loan forgiveness is a taxable event, so you will owe extra taxes in later years on money previously earned—and prob-ably already spent.

There are lenders that specialize in medical practice purchase and start-up, and offer up to 100% financing, including living expenses, including Bank of America Practice Solutions and Wells Fargo Practice Finance.

One of the most common mistakes I see doctors make in starting a practice is wasting time worrying about the wrong things in advance. Get a general overview by reading one or more of the "startup" books or articles, then get an expert startup consultant to customize the overload of information to your particular situation. For example, you can easily spend 100 hours studying just EMRs, when an expert consult might narrow down the choices to one or two within minutes. You can spend hours crafting a chart of accounts with an inexperienced CPA, when there are just two national standards you should choose-from: MGMA's and NSCHBC's.

Startup consultants can be found nationwide through their professional association, the National Society of Certified Healthcare Business Consultants (NSCHBC. org), whose members specialize in solo and small group practices, and from organizations like MGMA and AGMA, which specialize in larger group practices.

A high percentage of doctors end up in practice either near their hometown-, in an area similar to where they grew up, or near their family or family of their spouse. If you are considering setting up practice in a place very different from one of those scenarios, and if there is a question as to whether you will like your locale, you should rent an office and home for the first few years rather than buying or building one, just in case you end up leaving.

Try to find an existing office to fit your practice into without having to add leasehold improvements like a full interior.

You can sometimes convert regular CPA-type offices into medical spaces by using fully contained mobile sink units with a 5-gallon water source and 5-gallon waste container built in, expanding your options into atypical locations. If you have to pay for full leasehold improvements, plan on staying in that office at least 10 years to amortize that extra cost.

Before buying the real estate, get a good financial-planning consult from your CPA or financial planner. (This is discussed in Chapter 5.) Being your own tenant has some advantages, but it also puts your real estate investment into the same "risk basket" as your profession. If you become personally disabled or deceased, you or your estate then have the risk of losing your "tenant" and your real estate investment along with your professional income. If there is no office available to rent and you must build, consider building a four-plex office instead of just a solo office, and be sure to use an experienced medical-office architect. Rent the three other offices to complementary specialties to further diversify your risk and increase referrals, such as to a dentist, a chiropractor, a pharmacy, a lab or imaging center, or CPA. Then, if you become disabled, you still have three other tenants in other fields covering the mortgage.

One group of 10 savvy physician investors I know formed a real estate investment club into which they each contribute $100,000 per year. They use the $1 million to buy distressed commercial properties (never medical) for cash, to diversify their investment portfolios away from their profession, reducing overall portfolio risk. They are smart enough to not own their own offices!

Many physicians are moving into one of the types of "concierge" practices, including direct care, cash, retainer-with-insurance, and retainer-without-insurance. In most cases, I recommend a physician not create a concierge practice from scratch, but instead build (or buy) a typical insurance-based practice for a year or two, then convert to concierge so that an opportunity was maximized to build patient relationships that will withstand the conversion.

Most practices switching to concierge lose at least half to two-thirds of their patients when they make the transition. It's still easier than trying to attract concierge patients from scratch, unless the market is significantly underserved, such that patient-waits for appointments are measured in months rather than weeks or days.

As an alternative to concierge practice, there are more opportunities for practices to be "out of network" except perhaps for a few of the best insurance plans. Those "out of network" patients pay your full fee and submit your fees to their own insurance plans for reimbursement. Consider building a full-insured practice, then go out of network on few of the worst plans each year until some balance is achieved. Concierge practice is not necessarily a means to wealth. Most of the concierge physicians I know earn equal to or less than their insurance-based peers, but have a more satisfactory professional life.

As a physician, there will frequently be a career opportunity to start a practice, even though it might be non-traditional, like doing a "non-boarded specialty" (a family practitioner limiting their practice to dermatology), one of the versions of concierge medicine, or alternative or complimentary medicine. Get professional help, don't try to do it on your own, and you should be either fine, or having avoided a mistake.

SUMMARY

In summary, there are many ways to start a medical career. First decide where you would like to practice, do a little research on community need, then look around for available options and support resources. One way or another–with a little bit of thought and planning–you can hardly avoid being successful.

Resources

NSCHBC.org for consultants and lawyers, and practice income and expense statistics reports

MGMA.com for compensation and productivity data on jogs

Bank of America's or Wells Fargo's healthcare divisions for loans

Greenbranch.com for books on practice management and finance

Salary.com for job descriptions and compensation data for employing support staff

References

1. 2015 Survey of Final-Year Medical Residents. MerrittHawkins.com.
2. Medical School Applicants, Enrollment Reach All-time Highs. AAMC. September 2013.
3. 2014 Outlook on Health Care Providers. Deloitte.com.
4. Using Payments to Drive Cost-reducing Innovations. *Health International.* McKinsey's Healthcare Systems and Services Practice, 2012.
5. Health Law to Raise Costs. *AP.* March 27, 2013.
6. What Issues Will Most Affect Physicians in 2013? AAFP. January 7, 2013.
7. Doctors Have To Take a Pay Cut Under ObamaCare. *Forbes.* June 28, 2013.
8. BlueShieldCA.com.
9. Network Squeeze, Modern Healthcare. McKinsey & Co.
10. Surviving in a Network. MGMA *e-Source.* Reprinted in February 11, 2014.
11. DaVita HealthCarePartners.com.
12. Will ACOs Increase the Value of Your Practice? David Kibbe MD, AAFP Chair Senior Advisor.
13. MinuteClinic Acquired by CVS. CVSHealth.com. September 20, 2014.
14. MerchantMedicine.com and PBS.org and *Medical Economics* Aug 14, 2014

CHAPTER 4

Understanding and Negotiating Physician Employment Agreements

Thomas Shapira, Esq.

THE NEED FOR PHYSICIANS TO UNDERSTAND the issues that arise during the process of negotiating an employment agreement is critical. Whether coming out of a residency or a fellowship, or having been in practice and starting a new position, physicians must ensure that the employment contract adequately protects their rights and reflects the intention of the parties.

Many physicians, intimidated by a lengthy agreement full of legalese, may be inclined to simply scan the document for a few highlights rather than conducting a thorough review. Even if an employer provides a prospective physician with the employer's "standard" agreement and insists that it cannot be negotiated, the physician must still understand the impact of all of the provisions and, when necessary, attempt to negotiate the terms. For the remainder of this chapter, we will refer to the prospective physician employee as the "Physician" and the employer, whether a private practice or hospital/health system, as the "Practice"

INITIAL DUE DILIGENCE

Before doing an initial review of the agreement, the Physician should consider whether he or she trust the owners of the Practice. Such trust may be discerned from visits to the Practice and discussions with other physicians in the Practice, as well as with other physicians in the Practice's community. No employment agreement can cover every potential eventuality in the relationship between the Physician and the Practice, and if the Physician does not have an underlying level of trust that the Practice will be fair and equitable in interpreting the contract, problems are certain to arise.

It also is important that the Physician have a sense of how the Practice is run and whether it fits the Physician's own style of practice. Will the Physician be expected to assume significant call responsibilities and/or research projects? Does the Practice encourage a sense of collegiality among its physicians? Will the Physician be expected to see a high volume of patients? The Physician must speak with both the owners of the Practice and the other employed physicians to get a full sense of what will be expected. In the course of this "due diligence" of the Practice, the Physician should also inquire about the Practice's malpractice claim history to determine whether a pending matter may have a serious impact on the Practice's viability going forward.

Finally, the Physician should try to gauge his or her ability to negotiate the proposed employment agreement. Even a "standard" form may be subject to some modification, whether with respect to compensation, bonus thresholds, tail responsibility, paid time off, time to partnership, or restrictive covenants. The Physician may learn that one or more of these specific business terms vary among employed physicians at the Practice.

COMPENSATION

For many physicians, the most important provision of the employment agreement addresses compensation. Compensation may be a fixed annual amount, subject to increase, or it may be a percentage of receipts attributable to the Physician's professional services. In a percentage-based arrangement, the percentage retained by the Practice is roughly the equivalent of the overhead attributable to the Physician, and also likely includes some profit margin for the Practice. To the extent the Practice is a hospital and not a private group, regulatory restrictions prohibit compensation in excess of the fair market value of the Physician's services. Fair market value is represented by a range, not a specific point, and will vary based on the location of the Practice, the Physician's specialty, and how the Physician's workload differs from that of other similarly situated physicians (e.g., total work relative value units, or wRVUs).

If the Physician is moving to the Practice's community, the Practice may pay a relocation bonus, whether in the form of a pre-established stipend or reimbursement up to some certain amount. Occasionally, a Practice may pay a signing bonus. In addition to base compensation, the employment agreement may provide for an annual bonus. Specifics of such a bonus may be vague, providing for some bonus only at the discretion of the Practice. The Physician should negotiate this provision to provide more certainty as to the standards used to determine such a bonus.

Frequently, a bonus will be some percentage of the total annual receipts attributable to the Physician's professional services in excess of a pre-determined threshold. The threshold ensures that the Practice has covered all of its expenses attributable to the Physician, including compensation and the cost of Physician's benefits, as well as some profit for the Practice. As a result, the threshold may be between two and three times the Physician's base compensation amount. The Physician should ensure that the bonus amount will be prorated for any partial year that the Physician is employed by the Practice.

The employment agreement should address the Physician's ability to moonlight and/or engage in non-clinical activities, specifying permitted activities and how revenue from such activities will be treated (e.g., whether to be retained by the Physician or by the Practice). If the Physician knows certain activities in which she intends to participate (e.g., medical-legal consulting, teaching, medical directorships, outside research, authoring books/articles), those activities should be identified in the agreement.

TERM/TERMINATION

The employment agreement will specify the term of employment and may include renewal terms. The Physician must understand whether such renewals will occur automatically, or if the parties must take action at the end of the then-current term in order to renew. Many contracts include a provision for termination without cause. Such a provision is a double-edged sword for the Physician. On the one hand, it provides the Physician with the opportunity to terminate the agreement for any reason. On the other hand, the Practice also has the ability to terminate without cause.

The Physician must recognize that if the contract allows for termination by either party without cause on 120 days' notice, a five-year contract is in reality only a four-month agreement. The Practice will probably not agree to remove such a provision. Although seemingly allowing the Practice to terminate the Physician in an arbitrary manner, the real benefit to the Practice of such a provision is that it avoids a dispute with a difficult physician related to a "for-cause" termination, and can thereby avoid an extended negotiation (or even litigation) in order to achieve the termination. Especially if a Physician is relocating, it is reasonable that the Physician would insist that if the "without-cause" termination provision cannot be deleted, neither party can trigger that provision prior to the completion of the first year of the agreement. In that way, the Physician can be secure in the knowledge that there is, at a minimum, one year of job security.

The agreement will allow termination by the Practice for cause. "For-cause" events may include loss of state medical license, exclusion from the Medicare or Medicaid programs, inability to be insured, substance abuse, conduct harmful to the Practice's patients or the Practice's reputation, a felony conviction, or termination of the Physician's hospital medical staff membership or privileges.

The Physician should insist on receiving notice from the Practice of any alleged breach and, depending on the basis for the termination, an opportunity to "cure" the issue. Loss of license or insurance or exclusion from Medicare may not be curable offenses. However, more subjective termination criteria, such as failure to follow the policies of the Practice or even a temporary suspension of hospital privileges, may be cured and the Physician should insist on an opportunity to do so.

Similarly, the Physician should have the ability to terminate the agreement for cause. The most likely "cause" for the Physician would be if the Practice fails to pay the Physician in a timely manner. The basis for termination may impact other provisions, such as application of the restrictive covenant and/or an obligation to pay for tail coverage, as discussed later.

The agreement should also provide for termination in the event of a change of law that impacts the employment relationship. Change of law provisions allow the parties to attempt to negotiate an amendment to avoid any new legal issues, while preserving the parties' original economical intent. If such negotiation does not result in a mutually agreeable amendment, the parties have the ability to terminate.

The agreement should address whether the Physician will be entitled to any severance upon termination. If the Physician's compensation is a percentage of receipts, the termination provision should include a right to compensation for receipts attributable to services rendered prior to the termination date, but collected by the Practice after the termination date.

INSURANCE

Another important section of the employment agreement will address professional liability insurance coverage for the Physician. This provision should specify minimum coverage limits, often based on what is required by the medical staff bylaws of the applicable hospital. In addition, the provision should specify that the coverage for the Physician will be in the same amounts as provided to other physicians by the Practice. Usually, the Practice is responsible for paying the premiums for this coverage, but if the Physician is an independent contractor (rather than an employee), the Physician would be responsible for the premiums.

Coverage may be on a "claims-made" or an "occurrence" basis. Claims-made coverage applies only when the Physician is covered under the policy at the time the actual claim is made. An occurrence policy covers claims arising out of conduct that occurred while the Physician was employed by the Practice, even if such claim is made after the Physician has left the Practice.

Another issue related to professional liability coverage has to do with extended or tail coverage that insures the Physician for claims attributable to the period during which the Physician was employed by the Practice, even if such claims are not brought until the Physician is no longer with the Practice. Tail coverage is necessary only if the underlying policy is a claims-made policy. The cost of tail coverage may be high, so responsibility for the premiums for this coverage is often negotiated. Typically, that responsibility lies with the Physician, but the Practice may assume responsibility for that liability to the extent the Practice terminates the Physician without cause, or if the Physician is forced to terminate the agreement as a result of a breach by the Practice (e.g., with cause termination).

The flip-side of tail coverage is "nose" coverage, which applies to claims arising from the Physician's professional services before the start of the employment term. Nose coverage may not be necessary if the Physician was previously covered under an occurrence policy. Often, physicians coming out of residency or fellowships are covered by the hospital's policies, which are usually occurrence-based.

BENEFITS

The contract will identify the benefits available to Physician, specifying the permitted personal time (e.g., vacation, sick, etc.) to which the Physician is entitled, which may increase annually. The Physician should clarify whether unused time rolls over to future years, or if the Practice's policy is "use it or lose it." The agreement should also specify the amount of time available to the Physician for continuing medical education activities, in addition to any other vacation, personal, or sick time. If the agreement addresses time off as a result of disability, it should also be clear as to the compensation and benefits that will be paid during all or a portion of any such disability.

The Physician should understand what expenses will be paid directly by the Practice or will be reimbursed to the Physician, and if there is a cap on such amounts. The Physician should carefully review a list and description of benefits that are provided to similarly situated employees of the Practice, including health and any other insurance, as well as any pension program. Although the benefits may be amended from time to time over the course of the agreement, the Physician will want the Practice to agree that any amendment will apply to all the Practice's employees, and not single out the Physician.

RESTRICTIVE COVENANTS

One of the most important provisions of an employment agreement relates to restrictive covenants that limit the Physician's ability to practice medicine in the community following termination of the employment agreement. The enforceability of restrictive covenants is governed by state law. In most states, restrictive covenants are enforceable with respect to a physician if the covenant is reasonable in scope and duration, and does not unreasonably prohibit the Physician from earning a living.

A "reasonable" scope and duration is based on many factors, including the specific area in which the Practice is located. In the middle of a large metropolitan area, the geographic scope of an enforceable restrictive covenant is likely more limited in order to prevent foreclosing the Physician from numerous opportunities. Conversely, in a rural area, the scope may be significant if there are no other providers within close proximity. Enforceability is evaluated by most courts on a case-by-case basis. The Physician should attempt to speak to other employed physicians in the Practice to find out the scope of the Practice's "standard" restrictive covenant and to get a sense of what the Practice is willing to negotiate.

To the extent that the Physician is being recruited to the Practice through a not-for-profit hospital, federal regulation will prohibit a covenant that restricts the Physician from continuing to practice medicine in the community. In those situations, it is likely that the covenants will consist only of a non-solicitation of the Practice's patients and/or employees. The Physician should expect such a non-solicitation to be standard in the employment agreement, along with covenants related to confidentiality and nondisclosure of the Practice's patient and business information.

Similar to the negotiation of tail coverage, the Physician should consider negotiating application of the restrictive covenant. Typically, such covenants apply upon termination of the employment agreement for any reason, but the Physician may negotiate this provision to specifically not apply in the event the Physician is forced to terminate the agreement for cause, or the Practice terminates the employment agreement without cause.

PARTNERSHIP OR OTHER OWNERSHIP

One consideration for the Physician will be the possibility of ownership of the Practice, whether as a partner of a partnership, a shareholder of a corporation, or a member of a limited liability company. The Physician should understand the tax and liability implications of ownership of the applicable entity, which differ from those of an employee. Even if the Practice is not guaranteeing any future ownership, the Physician should inquire about how potential ownership would occur and what criteria the Practice will use in making such a determination.

Questions related to the effect of ownership on Physician's compensation, timing of such a decision, the formula for the buy-in amount that the Physician will be expected to pay, and the terms of such payment are all legitimate questions. Many practices will specifically not guarantee a right to ownership, but may indicate when the Practice expects such decision to be considered or made.

MISCELLANEOUS

Patient records generated by the Physician will be the property of the Practice, but the agreement should grant the Physician access to those records following termination of employment for purposes of any litigation, governmental audit, or billing investigation. The agreement should also specify the locations at which the Physician will render services, whether specific office locations and/or hospitals. If the Practice anticipates expanding, it may be unwilling to limit the Physician's services to those specific locations; however, the Physician should negotiate that any additional Practice locations will be mutually agreed upon.

For hospitals at which the Physician is required to be on staff, as well as managed care contacts to which the Physician will be subject, the Practice should be responsible for credentialing the Physician at the Practice's expenses. The Physician will be required to comply with all Practice policies, procedures, and rules, but the Physician needs to have some idea what those policies, procedures, and rules will be. Ideally, the contract will specify that the Physician is obligated to comply with those policies only to the extent they are made available to him or her.

Finally, the employment agreement should require the Practice to provide all facilities, supplies, and personnel reasonably necessary for the Physician's medical practice. If the Physician and the Practice have discussed specific needs for the Physician, such as an exclusive medical assistant or registered nurse, or some particular equipment or technology, the employment agreement must specify what will be provided.

USE OF LEGAL COUNSEL

Although the various items in this chapter will help the Physician read, understand, and negotiate an employment agreement, it is no substitute for retaining legal counsel. Experienced healthcare counsel may be more expensive than an attorney in general practice (e.g., similar to a specialist and an internist), but the legal rights and obligations of the Physician at stake in such an agreement justifies the expense. Too many physicians attempt to shortcut this process and not use counsel, or rely on the Practice's "standard" form of employment agreement, only to discover later that the Physician does not have the rights he or she expected, or has become bound by unexpected obligations that may adversely impact his or her future Practice.

It is also important for the Physician to control the relationship with counsel. The Physician should be active in this relationship, asking numerous questions in order to fully understand the issues, as well as demanding a high quality of service and responsiveness, both to the Physician and to the Practice's counsel. Legal counsel will advise the Physician of the various issues to protect the Physician's rights, but ultimately the Physician must decide if the particular relationship with the Practice is desirable in light of the terms of the employment agreement and how the provisions of that document may affect the Physician's medical practice going forward.

This chapter addresses the various provisions a Physician can expect to encounter in an employment agreement with a prospective employer. The Physician needs to understand the function of each provision and how it will impact the Physician's employment relationship and medical practice. In addition, the Physician should recognize options for negotiating those provisions to reduce the Physician's risk and maximize the Physician's benefit from such a relationship. Importantly, such an understanding is no substitute for representation by experienced legal counsel who can guide the Physician through such negotiation and ensure that the Physician does not run afoul of the many regulatory hurdles that can arise in the context of medical practice or hospital employment.

CHAPTER 5

Establishing Your Legal and Financial Teams and Setting Priorities

Joel M. Blau and Ronald J. Paprocki

PHYSICIANS ASK US FOR GUIDANCE in any number of areas, yet they all seem to relate to independence—the ability to do what you want—and dignity—the ability to do what you want in the *manner you wish*. Both of these elements are critical for a financially successful future.

Independence and dignity cannot easily be achieved without careful planning and execution, as well as time for implementation. The financial plan cannot be put into place in just a day.

Some physicians believe independence and dignity are achieved only through financial means. Not true! The financial aspect certainly plays a very important part, but there is more to independence and dignity than money. The process begins with goals relating to future income, lifestyles, and experiences. Often, goals relating to personal relationships become the foundation of success.

A financial plan is imperative to accomplishing independence and dignity and to reaching short- and long-term objectives. Coordinating these important components of the decision-making process can mean the difference between a successful, happy life and an unhappy, unfulfilling future. The consequences associated with poor planning can leave you financially strained and not able to reach your goals. To be flexible in an ever-changing profession, you need to gain knowledge of the financial planning process and use it as a road map going forward.

The first step in creating a financial plan is developing a series of short-term and long-term goals and objectives, such as buying a home, financing a college education for your children, or enjoying your ultimate retirement. A properly structured financial plan also will address the areas of life over which we have little control, such as death and disability.

Next, you are ready to create the financial tool that is a mainstay of financially successful physicians. It is exciting, thought-provoking and stimulating: it's a budget! Budgets may be boring, but they are necessary; otherwise, you put yourself at a financial disadvantage.

Compile a list of your assets and liabilities, your income and expenditures. There are a number of ways to track income and expenditures. Some traditional methods are paper based; a number are available online. Without a budget, you have no real sense of what you need to do or how to get there. This is a basic but critically important process to complete.

Now, identify financial advisors who may be a part of your team. When you completed your residency, the first financial advisor to contact you probably was not an advisor but an insurance agent. The agent probably talked about the effect your premature death or disability would have on your family and told you that your most important asset was your ability to earn income, so you must insure against its loss. Here the solutions are often times leading to the purchase of life and disability insurance, especially early in your career. (For more, see Chapter 6.)

Another potential advisor is an attorney, who can address the concept of hazard protection—estate planning. Regardless of your income or the size of your estate, you must make decisions today that will affect your family tomorrow. You want to make certain your plan is successful even if you are not around to witness it! If you have children, you must name guardians and trustees and detail how assets should be treated upon your death. (More estate planning alternatives are provided in Chapter 6.)

After setting down a solid foundation, build a layer of cash reserves for emergencies, such as car repair, roof repair, or a month when expenses exceed income. Cash reserves include assets that do not fluctuate in value and are available and liquid when you need them. The risk/reward tradeoff for cash reserves is that these low-risk vehicles usually provide the lowest interest rates and thus do not offer meaningful growth potential. An emergency reserve is necessary since the worst time to sell any investment is when you are forced to convert the asset to cash.

Financial planning practitioners recommend that an emergency fund should equal approximately three times your monthly living expenses. This is an adequate amount assuming your income is predictable and consistent. If, on the other hand, you are a sole practitioner and your monthly income is more erratic, you may want to have as much as six times your average monthly total living expenses allocated to cash equivalents.

To determine an appropriate funding level, take a close look at your average monthly living expenses (your standard of living) as identified in the budget you developed. Total all the checks you wrote during a one-month period. Use two or three months to get a better idea of your average monthly expenses. Don't forget to include a portion of large bills that may be paid only yearly, such as insurance premiums, property taxes, and home improvements.

After you've created an emergency fund, you can move on to investing in liquid investments that have the potential for greater-than-bank's rate of return. Liquid investments will show some fluctuation of principal. For example, at the time of sale, the value of a liquid investment asset can be more or less than the original investment. Examples of liquid investments are stocks, bonds, or mutual funds and exchange traded funds (ETFs) that invest in stocks or bonds. Also included are cash values of variable-life insurance policies.

Unlike cash reserves, liquid investments have the potential to earn higher returns over time. But along with this comes value fluctuation or risk. In general, there is nothing wrong with taking on increased risk, as long as you have an adequate emergency fund to provide the needed protection for your cash flow needs.

Other types of investments are longer term and less liquid. Examples of longer-term investments are qualified retirement plans, including pension and profit-sharing plans, self-employed plans (SEPs), simple plans, and individual retirement accounts (IRAs)—both traditional as well as the Roth IRA. The investments in these plans may be cash equivalents, stocks, bonds, mutual funds, or other types of investments. As a general rule, consider these funds to be illiquid until you reach age 59½. Withdrawals from these plans before age 59½ are typically assessed with a 10% IRS penalty and constitute taxable income in the year received.

DEBT REDUCTION

As you consider your financial future at the beginning of your career, you will need to make decisions relative to your debt. The term "debt" simply means anything you owe to another entity. The most common types of debt for physicians at the beginning of their careers are student loans and credit card debt. With respect to student loans, it makes sense to have your financial advisor help you create a strategy to pay off the loans. This will be a function of your income, current level of debt, as well as the interest rates associated with the debt.

From an analytical standpoint, a number of "what if" scenarios can be calculated to determine if it makes the most sense to pay off debts as quickly as possible or spread out the payments to allow you to invest in potentially appreciating assets at the same time. But that is the analytical solution, not necessarily a personal, emotional decision. You must look beyond the numbers to determine your own debt-comfort level.

Some physicians may want to pay off the loans as soon as possible so they have a comfortable peace of mind about their financial situation, while others are more than content to pay off the loans as slowly as possible. The answer for you rests with your ability to look forward toward your other longer-term financial goals to determine a payoff strategy that makes the most sense for your own situation.

Loan consolidation programs have fallen out of favor over the past years but are beginning to make a comeback. Consider this alternative, especially if you are committed to building wealth in a variety of areas and are willing to balance the potential of higher investment returns compared to fixed interest rate payments.

This theory, though, does not apply to credit card debt. Credit card interest rates are higher relative to other forms of debt and offer no tax advantages. Be certain that you are living within your means and not spending money on luxury items that you may not be able to afford. In the perfect world, all purchases made during the month should be paid off in full every billing cycle. If this is not happening, then you are probably spending money that you do not have, thus living beyond your means. This is not a healthy situation, and if it has been a habit of yours during your early years, now is the time to focus on controlling your spending. Quite simply, you will not be in the best position to achieve future savings goals if all of your excess funds are going toward loan repayments. Typically, the best scenario is to pay off credit card debt as soon as possible so that those future savings dollars can be redirected to a more efficient manner of systematic savings.

INCOME AND INTEREST

Many investment vehicles have an income component. Income can be derived from interest (bank savings accounts, certificates of deposit, and bonds), dividends (common stock and mutual funds), or capital gains distributions (mutual funds). In the case of bank accounts and mutual funds, you have the option of getting the income in the form of a check every month (or whenever distributed), or reinvesting the income back into the original investment. The latter is referred to as compounding.

If you are in need of current income, you have no choice but to receive an income distribution. On the other hand, if you do not currently need the income, you should consider compounding. Compounding can affect your actual returns in a positive way. Consider for a moment a $100,000 bank CD paying an annual interest rate of 3%. If you choose to take the income as a monthly distribution, you will receive $3,000 per year ($100,000 x 3%), or $250 per month. If, on the other hand, you choose to compound each month (interest is left in the investment), you will annually earn $3,041.60. This in effect represents a yield of

3.042%. At the end of 10 years (ignoring taxes for the moment), this CD would be worth $134,392.

Interestingly, if you were to double the rate of return to 6%, taken as a distribution, the annual income would be $6,000. If the amount were left to compound monthly, the actual dollar return would be $6,167.78—an effective yield of 6.167%. The value of the CD after 10 years would be approximately $179,085.

Compounding allows your investment dollars to work for you instead of you working to save even more. As a general rule, if you don't need the current income generated by your investments, don't take it—let it compound.

RETIREMENT PLANNING: 401(K)/403(B)

Unfortunately, many physicians forget the importance of compounding in their retirement years. During their working years, they compound simply because earned income satisfies their spending needs. At retirement, they contact their brokers and investment managers and instruct them to turn on the faucet and let the income flow. But what if there is more income than the retiree needs? This extra money is no longer affected by the exponential relationship of compounding. The key is to remove only that income that is needed.

401(k) Plans

Younger physicians should take advantage of employer-sponsored retirement plans. Internal Revenue Code Section 401(k) retirement savings programs allow employees to contribute on their own behalf, on a pre-tax basis, with the benefit of tax-deferred compounding similar to traditional IRAs, pension, and profit-sharing plans. The maximum allowable pre-tax contribution for employees is $18,000 for 2016. Employees age 50 and over may be able to contribute an additional $6,000 via the "catch up deferral." The plan may also include a 401(k) Roth provision allowing the employee to make after-tax contributions. Based on current tax law, Roth contributions are made with after-tax dollars but are received on a tax-free basis at retirement.

For physicians to be able to contribute the maximum allowable amount to their 401(k) plans, there also must be participation from the lower-compensated employees to ensure that the plan is not discriminatory.

A traditional 401(k) plan is subject to two nondiscrimination tests: the actual deferral percentage (ADP) test for employee elective deferrals, and the actual contribution percentage (ACP) test for matching contributions. Now as an alternative, an employer may adopt a "safe harbor" 401(k) plan, which is not subject to nondiscrimination testing.

Under current tax law, there are two safe harbor alternatives to the ADP test. In the first, the employer makes a non-elective contribution of 3% to each eligible highly compensated and non-highly compensated employee. The other alternative offers the employer the opportunity to make matching contributions of 100% of non-highly compensated employee elective contributions up to 3% of pay, and 50% of non-highly compensated employee additional elective contributions up to 5% of pay. All matches and non-elective contributions made to satisfy the safe harbor must be immediately vested. In addition, the employer must notify employees within a reasonable period of time, prior to the plan year, of their rights and obligations under the safe harbor arrangement.

By meeting the above criteria, many highly compensated owner/physicians will find they actually will be able to accrue a greater benefit for themselves. With the objective of most qualified retirement plans being tax-advantaged growth for future income needs, obviously the greater amount allowed to be invested annually can make a dramatic difference down the road. Often acting as contribution limitations, guidelines are in place to ensure that there is not a great disparity of contributions, with highly compensated key employees receiving the lion's share. The "safe harbor" alternative to the traditional 401(k) plan will enable many physicians to accrue a greater retirement benefit while still conforming to IRS guidelines. Based on the history of prior employee participation, the safe harbor plan may prove to be a viable alternative for those wanting to maximize their retirement planning options.

Not surprisingly, financial independence remains a primary goal for most physicians. While the desirability of this goal hasn't changed over the years, the feasibility of attaining it has. Faced with lower incomes and longer hours, physicians will come to rely more heavily on their portfolio returns, especially within qualified retirement plans, in order to become financially independent. Whether an owner or an employee, physicians may be able to become involved in investment decisions to better fit their long-term personal objectives.

403(b) Plans

The 403(b) is a tax-deferred retirement plan, similar to the 401(k) plan, but available only to employees of public educational institutions and some nonprofit (tax-exempt) organizations.

Unlike the 401(k), the 403(b) is not required to abide by Employee Retirement Income Security Act (ERISA) rules, even though many consider it a "qualified" plan. Like 401(k) plans, 403(b) plans have the standard penalty-free distribution age of 59½, but with an exception: if the employee separates from services in the year he or she is turning 55 and is considered retired, there will be no early 10% withdrawal penalty.

403(b) plans are similar to 401(k) plans in that the investment earnings grow tax-deferred until withdrawal, at which time they are taxed as ordinary income. 403(b) plans may also include a 403(b) Roth provision allowing employee after-tax contributions. Employers are allowed to match the total contributions the employee makes into both plans, but will be able to only deposit matches into the traditional (non-Roth) 403(b) account. Maximum allowable pre-tax contributions are the same as 401(k) plans.

CHILDREN'S EDUCATION

Saving for a college education is one of the most daunting financial tasks a family can face, requiring as much commitment and careful planning as arranging your own retirement plan and your estate.

But a powerful tool can enable you to put aside money for your family members' educations as well as reduce your estate tax exposure. The Section 529 plan, named after the section of the Internal Revenue Code authorizing it, allows you to remove wealth from your estate while you steadily accumulate assets to help educate children, grandchildren, nieces, nephews—and even yourself, if you're planning to go back to college.

These accounts are particularly useful for grandparents looking for ways to limit the tax hit on a lifetime of assets. You can set up accounts for several grandchildren and reap the same rewards from each account. While Section 529 accounts are usually set up for children and grandchildren, no family relationship is required. You can set up an account for any college-bound student you want to help.

There are big tax advantages to Section 529 college savings accounts. Briefly, these state-sponsored accounts are allowed to accumulate earnings free of any federal income tax (usually free of state income tax too). Then, when the account beneficiary reaches college age, tax-free withdrawals can be taken to pay for the beneficiary's qualified college expenses.

Section 529 plans accept large lump-sum contributions (over $200,000 in most cases), creating a unique opportunity to reduce the taxable estate. For federal gift tax purposes, the contributions are treated as completed gifts eligible for the annual gift tax exclusion of $14,000 for 2016. You can elect to spread a lump-sum contribution over five years and thereby immediately benefit from five years' worth of annual federal gift tax exclusions. You make the election on the federal gift tax return. However, if you die during the five-year spread period, a pro-rata portion of the contribution is added back to your estate for federal estate tax purposes.

While many savings incentive plans limit participation based on annual earnings, the Section 529 plan is available to all taxpayers regardless of their income. The investor receives the advantages of tax-free buildup and withdrawal, limited control over the funds invested, and no restrictions as to the school attended, as long as the money is used for higher education. Section 529 savings plans do not offer a guarantee that the funds accumulated will be sufficient to pay future education costs; whatever the fund grows to is what will be available.

The various state plans offer many investment options based on the amount of risk an investor wants to take. Many states also offer plans designed around the child's age, typically becoming more conservative as the child approaches college age.

Almost all states offer their own Section 529 plan, which is managed by an investment management company chosen by each state. While the IRS permits tax-free buildup as well as withdrawals, a state can add its own perks, such as state tax deductions on deposits. However, if funds are not withdrawn to pay higher education expenses, the taxpayer must pay tax on the gains in addition to a 10% IRS penalty. This situation can be avoided by using the remaining funds for other family members (such as siblings), under the same criteria.

While the basic features of Section 529 plans are mighty attractive, physicians may realize substantial benefits that have nothing to do with saving for college education costs. One of the major non-tax-related advantages of the Section 529 plan pertains to control. As opposed to Uniformed Gift to Minors accounts (UGMA) or Uniform Transfer to Minors accounts (UTMA) where the minor takes ownership of the account once he or she reaches the age of majority, Section 529 plans allow the account owner, usually a parent or grandparent, to maintain full control of the assets as well as the timing of the distributions. The owner also has the right to change the beneficiary of the account at any time. Doing so creates no tax liability as long as the new beneficiary is a member of the previous beneficiary's family, which by definition includes parents, siblings, aunts, uncles, cousins, nieces, and nephews.

Also worth considering is the use of Section 529 plans as an asset-protection strategy. As these accounts grow in value, asset protection will become a higher priority, especially in light of judgments that go beyond malpractice insurance coverage limits. Please note, the ability of judgment creditors to reach Section 529 assets varies from state to state. This is especially important since donors are not mandated to use the plan offered through their own state. The restrictions do vary, with some states offering limited levels of protection. States with statutes restricting access by the donor's creditors obviously offer a greater level of asset protection.

If you are concerned about the Section 529 plan restricting your ability to obtain financial aid, calculating the impact is relatively simple when a parent is the owner of the Section 529 plan, because it is reported on the federal financial aid application (FAFSA) as a parental asset. This is something to consider when you take out a Section 529 plan. Schools individually set their own rules when determining need-based scholarships, and many schools are starting to adjust awards when they discover Section 529 plans in the family.

STARTING YOUR RETIREMENT PLAN

Many physicians find themselves unprepared for retirement, financially as well as emotionally. From the financial standpoint, the majority of physicians fail to reach their own financial objectives—as the saying goes, they don't plan to fail, they fail to plan.

The main reason physicians are not prepared for retirement is that they start saving too late and are unable to make up the shortfall during their peak earning years. This procrastination and poor planning can result in physicians having to continue to work in some manner during retirement or reduce the income desired during the retirement years.

Successful retirement planning requires three key elements:
1. Setting clear goals;
2. Maximizing tax benefits; and
3. Exercising discipline.

When setting a clear retirement goal, give thought to the age at which you would like to achieve financial independence—when you do not have to earn an income to support yourself. There is no better feeling than continuing to work on a full-time or part-time basis because you want to—not because you have to.

After you have determined the age at which you would like to achieve true financial independence, you will need to quantify the amount of income needed to maintain a comfortable standard of living. Rather than taking a generalized approach of targeting 70%–75% of your current standard of living, we recommend a more specific and personalized method of determination by spending the appropriate amount of time developing a budget. Consider which expenses you won't have or that will be less during retirement, and also think about categories of expenses that may increase, such as travel and other leisure activities. Next, take an inventory of your investment assets, including your retirement plans. What types of rates of return have you been earning and what can you expect in the future? Is your rate of inflation assumption realistic?

Exercising discipline makes the difference between financial independence security and failure. All the retirement and tax planning strategies in the world will prove ineffective if you don't actually implement a retirement planning strategy. You not only need to gather information and determine objectives, you need to make informal decisions and act on them. Don't put it off, as the sooner you begin, the greater the chance of enjoying a financially successful retirement.

Planning for retirement can be an enjoyable experience. Use the Checklist for Successful Retirement (see pg. 54) as a starting point.

SOCIAL SECURITY AND RETIREMENT

What benefits can you expect from your retirement plans? Should you count on Social Security? As you continue to pay into the Social Security system, you should be aware of the realities that face the future of the program.

Sixty years ago, there were approximately 42 workers contributing to the Social Security system for every retiree collecting a benefit. Today there are only 4 workers for every beneficiary. Projections indicate that by the year 2025, the ratio will have dropped to 2.2 workers per retiree. While legislators discuss various options to save the system, we can almost be assured that the outcome will involve higher taxes on working Americans, changes in accepted retirement ages, and lower benefits for at least some retirees.

In the past, when financial planning discussions turned to Social Security benefits, physicians with incomes in excess of $200,000 and million-dollar qualified retirement plans often discounted the need for Social Security benefits. The consensus was that with retirement plans and nonqualified savings growing exponentially, the need for government benefits was greatly reduced, if not eliminated. In addition, with retirement income goals in the six-figure range, many felt that even if Social Security benefits were available, the amount would barely make a dent in their standard of living. For physicians nearing retirement who have seen their retirement nest egg depleted by market forces, payments from Social Security play a far greater role in their annual retirement income needs.

Government figures suggest that unless changes are made, the system will run out of money. When the system runs out of money, and for the years to follow, the government will have to borrow money or raise taxes each and every year to pay the rising benefits. Unfortunately, many misconceptions exist about the workings of Social Security, and clarification of those points should better position you to proactively plan for your retirement income needs.

The first misconception is that the federal government saves or sets aside a portion of taxes collected to be used specifically for Social Security benefits. In reality, all of the tax dollars received by the government are spent quickly, typically in a matter of days.

Second, commonsense dictates that Social Security payroll taxes are earmarked for Social Security benefits. Commonsense, as many of you already realize, is not the government's modus operandi. The payroll taxes collected far exceed the amount required to pay the promised benefits. But the surplus is spent on other things completely unrelated to Social Security.

A close look at the numbers reveals a Social Security trust fund of approximately $1.2 trillion, which is expected to grow to $5 trillion by 2016. However, an even closer look reveals that the trust fund balance is a running tally of all the Social Security surplus money spent on other things over the years. That money is now gone. If, as anticipated, Social Security goes cash flow negative in a matter of years with no money in the trust fund, only IOUs, the government will need to borrow or raise taxes to redeem those IOUs and meet the anticipated shortfall.

This all leads to the premise that the Social Security trust fund contains real assets, which is certainly debatable. The reality is that the next generation may need to pay higher payroll taxes, perhaps high enough to fund half of an average retiree's benefit.

This does not bode well for those expecting to receive a certain Social Security retirement benefit. While Social Security was discounted in the past as an amount that would barely dent their retirement needs, newly retired physicians should take a closer look at the impact of the government benefits relative to their overall income needs and as a way to supplement income shortages during down cycles in the stock market. Younger practicing physicians may want to simply ignore the goings on of Social Security and instead save money at a greater pace and invest wisely in order to have greater control over their future financial security.

Lawmakers are weighing a number of proposals to deal with the fund's long-term solvency issues, including raising payroll taxes, increasing the amount of income subject to Social Security payroll taxes, raising the retirement age, or simply reducing future benefits. While there are quite a number of details and other options still to be considered, it does appear likely that some form of change in the Social Security system will need to take place.

Traditionally, the magic age to receive a full benefit was 65. Based on current law, for those born after 1937 but before 1960, the age of full retirement benefits is dependent on the specific year of birth. For those born in 1960 and later, full retirement benefits are payable at age 67. The benefit payable will, of course, be based on an individual's past earning record and is adjusted annually for inflation.

A reduced benefit remains available beginning at age 62. However, assuming a traditional current full retirement age (FRA) of 65, beginning benefits at age 62 reduces the monthly amount by 20%. With the new FRA, receiving an early benefit at age 62 would result in a monthly benefit reduction of approximately 30%. You can verify your FRA on the Retirement Age Calculator on the Social Security website (www.ssa.gov/pubs/ageincrease.htm).

In addition to deciding at which age to begin taking benefits, it is also important to understand how working affects your Social Security benefits. The Senior Citizens' Freedom to Work Act of 2000 repealed an earnings limitation on Social Security benefits for individuals ages 65 to 69. Under the current law, you generally can receive full Social Security benefits, regardless of earnings, starting with the month you reach FRA. If benefits are taken prior to the FRA, only $15,120 can be earned before a reduction in your Social Security benefits. Benefits are reduced by $1 for every $2 you earn above this amount.

Once benefits begin, earnings are defined as any wages earned as an employee and any net earnings from self-employment. Wages include bonuses, commissions, fees, vacation pay, and pay in lieu of vacation. Not included as earnings is investment income, including stock dividends, interest from savings accounts and CDs, annuity income, limited partnership income, and rental income from real estate. Also excluded from the earnings definition is income from Social Security, pensions or other retirement plan income, gifts, and inheritances.

While planning a strategy to maximize your Social Security benefits, the starting point is to ensure that all of your earnings are accurately recorded and to obtain an estimate of the amount of future benefits. The Social Security Administration (SSA) now automatically mails an annual benefit statement to each worker age 25 and older not receiving current benefits approximately one month prior to his or her birthday. You also may request the records at any time by completing form SSA-7004, "Request for Social Security Statement." The form can be requested by calling the SSA at 800–772–1213 or via the SSA website at www.ssa.gov.

CREATING AND USING AN INVESTMENT POLICY STATEMENT

While the current economic environment may seem different, there has historically been uncertainty in most, if not all, time periods. The key to determining what to invest in should be based primarily on the needs, temperament, and available resources of each individual or family. The best investment for one person is often far less suited for someone else. Advice given in the media or from others unfamiliar with your particular situation oftentimes adds to the confusion. That is why it's important to use an Investment Policy Statement (IPS). The IPS will outline what you are comfortable investing in and lay out the parameters for change and review. The process of choosing the most appropriate investment for your own specific situation can be made easier by carefully considering the following questions:

1. What are your investment goals? One way to look at this common question is to ask yourself, "What do I want my money to do for me?" For example, the investor who is a retiree might need additional income to meet current living expenses. Goals for working individuals may be longer term, such as saving for retirement, funding a child's education, financing a major purchase, or creating and maintaining an emergency fund.

2. How liquid does the investment need to be? The term "liquidity" refers to how quickly an investment can be turned into cash without losing any of the invested dollars, or principal. Investments designed to meet longer-term goals such as retirement generally do not need to be as liquid as those earmarked as emergency funds.

3. What is your risk tolerance? Can you afford to risk losing a portion or all of your investment without it affecting how you live? What would be the impact of a loss on your investment goals? In general, risk is related to return: the higher the risk, the higher the potential return; the lower the risk, the lower the potential return.

4. What is the impact of income taxes? Income taxes can have a significant negative impact on your investment results. For example, many high-income individuals invest in municipal bonds because the interest from such bonds is generally exempt from federal income tax, and in some instances the interest is also exempt from state income tax. Qualified retirement plans, life insurance policies, and annuity contracts are used to accumulate funds for retirement primarily because of their tax-advantaged nature.

5. What is the economic outlook? The state of the economy as a whole can cause investors to re-examine or change the mix of desired investments. For example, during periods of high inflation, tangible assets such as real estate and precious metals have tended to produce nice results. During periods of stable or declining inflation, intangible assets such as stocks and bonds have done generally well. But keep in mind; while this has been the case historically, there is no guarantee that history will repeat itself.

6. Is the skill and knowledge needed to manage the investment available? An investor may not have the specialized skills and knowledge needed to properly select or manage an investment. In such instances, professional investment advice, or investments where such advice is available, should be considered.

7. How much money is available to be invested? The investment tools open to an investor can vary, depending on the amount of money available. These questions are simply the starting point in developing an investment plan. By focusing on your own specific needs, goals and objectives, you can establish and maintain an efficient investment plan, even in periods of economic uncertainty.

Below is a checklist to help you plan for a successful retirement.

CHECKLIST FOR A SUCCESSFUL RETIREMENT

- Have your financial planner prepare a retirement income projection to ensure there are adequate assets to support your retirement standard of living.
- Anticipate and prepare for non-financial changes. After being with patients and colleagues for so long, many physicians miss the social aspect of medicine. One way around this is to work on a limited basis with shorter hours and no call. If you're interested in this kind of arrangement, explore the possibilities.
- While working a full schedule, have a business valuation conducted on your practice. This should provide a starting point for discussions about selling your share of the practice. Selling a practice may take upwards of two years.
- Determine liability coverage options and other asset-protection strategies to be used during retirement.
- Map out a strategy to coordinate the tax treatment of income generated from the rollover of qualified retirement plan assets.
- Decide who will assist you in managing your rollover portfolio during your retirement years.

CHAPTER 6

Insuring Your Future

Joel M. Blau and Ronald J. Paprocki

YOUNG PHYSICIANS APPROACH THEIR FIRST JOB in medicine in different
ways. Some are merely trying to gain experience and then plan to move
to another practice with that added training. Others join a practice with
the hope of establishing a long-term partnership relationship. Regardless of your
initial intent, that isn't always the final outcome due to changes initiated by the
practice ownership or by you. Still, it makes sense to ensure that you are well-
prepared financially in the event you leave your practice earlier than anticipated.

Beyond the legal questions relating to possible noncompete issues, there are three
important financial issues associated with leaving a practice early in your career:
how to ensure your future income in the event of a disability, how to guarantee
your family's financial well-being in the event of your death, and how to properly
move or transfer your retirement plan assets.

DISABILITY INSURANCE

Your most important asset is neither your home nor your investment account, but
your ability to earn future income. You have so much time and money invested
in your career that you simply cannot allow your income to unexpectedly stop—
which could happen if a disability renders you unable to work. Many practices
offer a group disability plan, but if you leave that practice, you may also be leaving
your coverage behind. If the new practice offers coverage, there may be a time gap
until the coverage becomes in force. In addition, the practices' plans may offer a
different level of benefits.

First, ask yourself if you are confident that your income is secure in the event of
disability. It is your responsibility as a young physician to take the lead in ensuring
that your future income will continue if you are disabled. Own your own policy,
select your benefit level, and maintain the policy regardless of future employment
changes. Preferring to accept the practice-provided plan, assuming that there is
one, regardless of the coverage amounts and definitions of disability, can be a
catastrophic mistake, jeopardizing you and your family's financial future. The

key is to gain an understanding of the disability insurance issues you are facing today and then ensure you are properly covered prior to making any job changes.

Unfortunately, a great number of plans may provide benefits substantially less than you would expect or that you will need should the situation of disability arise and you have to stop practicing medicine or significantly modify what your able to do.

The term "disability" can be defined in very different ways by the insurance company providing the plan. For example, one insurance carrier may provide benefits if you are "unable to perform the important duties of your profession and specialty." On the surface this sounds great in that this definition implies that if your occupation is limited to a recognized specialty, you will receive disability benefits even if you can continue working in another aspect of the medical profession. But you must read the fine print, and in this case, read the sentence that may follow the first definition. Often times the continued definition may state: "After two years [or five years in some policies] you must not be able to perform the duties of any occupation." So, if you can work in any job at all, medically based or not, you will not be considered "disabled" and your benefit payments will be discontinued.

It is clear why policies with this type of language are less costly than those that provide monthly benefits for as long as you are unable to work in your chosen field or specialty; the insurance company is assuming less risk. But are these policies really less expensive? If you continually pay your premiums but are denied benefits due to the limited definition of "disability" in the policy, it can ultimately cost you and your family substantially more.

The definition dilemma can occur in all types of disability coverage—group and association, as well as individually owned polices. Read the definition section of your current policy or any polices you may purchase in the future to ensure that your definition of "disability" is the same as that of the insurance company providing the coverage.

Other than the specific disability definition used within the policy, there are other important features and provisions that need to be examined and compared. "Partial" or "residual" disability benefits may be paid in some policies when the specific disability impairment allows the insured to perform only a portion of his or her duties. This provision may also pay benefits in the event the disability reduces the insured's income by a certain percentage of the pre-disability amount.

Another important provision deals with the ability to cancel and renew the policy. "Non-cancelable" generally means that the insurance company cannot cancel the policy, change the policy provisions, or increase the premiums after the policy is issued, and the premiums are paid on time. "Guaranteed renewable" is similar in all aspects, except that the insurance company has the ability to increase the premium amount. Another provision, typically added as an additional cost rider, is the cost of living adjustment (COLA). This rider provides the benefit of an inflation-adjusted monthly benefit, in the event of a disability claim, in order to keep pace with inflation. Some disability insurance policies increase by a fixed amount each year while others are indexed to inflation.

A COLA is of particular importance to young clients with longer life expectancies. For example, if a disability insurance policy paid an annual benefit of $100,000 for the first year for a total disability, and if a 3% compounded adjustment was applied for 20 years, the benefit amount after 20 years of total disability benefit would have grown to $180,611 for that year.

Of course, the more guaranteed provisions included in the policy, either as part of the original policy or as a rider, the higher the premium. Fortunately, there are a variety of ways to construct a policy so you have greater control over the ultimate premium amount. The first is the monthly amount of the benefit. Unfortunately, all disability insurance policies do not enable you to replace 100% of your income. Generally, you can purchase up to 60%–66% of your current income with a set dollar amount maximum, as the insurance companies do not want to give you an incentive to make a claim.

Next is the "waiting" and "elimination" period, which controls how long you must be disabled prior to receiving benefits, similar to a deductible but based on time, not dollars. Commonly available periods include 30, 60, 90, 180, and 360 days. Naturally, the longer the elimination period selected, the lower the premium payment amount will be. The key determinant will be your cash needs. For example, if you have a 90-day waiting period, you will need to maintain 3 months of cash reserves in the event of a disability. Also, we suggest that you take into account any other income sources available, such as a spouse's income, as well as the benefit period of any short-term disability coverage you may have through your practice.

The other major cost factor is the "benefit period." This will determine how long the benefits will be paid after the waiting or elimination period has been satisfied and the disability continues. Some companies offer lifetime benefits (the highest cost), but most provide benefits payable to age 65, benefits payable for five years, or shorter timeframes of 24 months (the lowest cost).

Clearly, there are many variables involved with structuring an efficient disability insurance program. The key is to work with an independent advisor who can show you various companies, options and their corresponding costs to ensure your future income in the event of a disability (see Chapter 12).

LIFE INSURANCE

Many physicians recognize the benefits of having an overall financial plan to meet their positive long-term objectives such as retirement planning, education planning, and long-term savings goals. However, planning for the unexpected via life insurance is certainly less pleasant and also quite difficult. Understandably, no one likes to contemplate their own demise, and there are so many other important issues that seem to take precedence over the life insurance decision-making process. Whatever the reason, delaying this important part of the planning process can result in expensive and unintended tragic consequences.

When planning for survivor income needs, you will need to consider the ongoing income needs of your survivors, as well as any immediate or short-term lump sum needs. First, determine how much income will be needed for the surviving family upon your death. Is the desire to maintain the current standard of living of the family, or will their needs be less? Will the family be staying in the same home or moving to a different location? Will the surviving spouse be earning income, or do you want to provide sufficient income so that the spouse will not need to generate income? From home mortgage standpoint, would you like to provide a lump sum payment for the balance of your home mortgage or other debt? With regard to college education funding, you will need to consider whether you prefer to leave a lump sum equal to the future college funding needs of your children.

These decisions are difficult but are important to quantifying life insurance needs. People buy life insurance when they do not have sufficient assets to provide for their survivors, so if you have sufficient investment assets to meet your survivor income objectives, there may not even be a need for life insurance. If you have sufficient assets, then you are considered to be self-insured. That's why oftentimes a physician's greatest need for life insurance is early in his or her career, prior to having saved substantial investment assets.

Many different types of life insurance products are available to meet the varying needs of physicians. Once you have defined the qualitative and quantitative need for life insurance, you can begin to determine which specific product in the life insurance marketplace best meets your objectives. The key, regardless of the reason you are buying life insurance, is to be certain that the specific life insurance product you are purchasing meets your unique objectives.

First, decide if your specific life insurance need is "temporary" or "permanent." Temporary would imply that your needs are relatively short-term. A good example would be if you are trying to provide survivor income in the event you die prior to becoming self-insured. Once you have accumulated sufficient assets to provide for your surviving family, you may no longer need the life insurance for that particular exposure. Permanent insurance, on the other hand, is generally purchased with the understanding that the policy proceeds will be paid out at the time of your death, regardless of when that occurs, even if you live beyond your expected mortality age.

Term Insurance

If your life insurance needs are temporary, term insurance may be the most appropriate vehicle to use. Term insurance has no cash value or savings component attached to it. Quite simply, you pay your premium, and if you die during that policy year, the death benefit is paid to your beneficiary. Decreasing term has a level premium, but a decreasing death benefit. It is generally used in conjunction with financial obligations that decrease over time, such as mortgages or other types of amortized loans.

Two types of term insurance offer a level death benefit, but a differing premium paying structure. Annual renewable term has a yearly increasing premium, which increases with the higher mortality cost associated with being a year older and a year closer to your expected mortality age. It is primarily used for financial obligations that remain constant for a relatively short period of time. Level premium term, on the other hand, offers a level premium payment amount over a fixed number of years, typically 5, 10, 15, or 20 years. This would be appropriate for needs that are finite in length, such as ensuring coverage until a young child has completed college, becoming self-insured through an increased net worth, or reaching retirement age with sufficient retirement income to meet your needs.

Other differences will be discovered when term policies are compared. The major areas impacting premium rates are policy provisions dealing with renewability and convertibility. Typically, renewable policies allow the policyholder the option of continuing term coverage after the stated period of time has expired. While the renewal will be at a higher premium rate than during the defined time period, new medical underwriting is not required. If during the term period, you become ill in a manner that would deem you to be uninsurable or insurable but with an added-on rating that would substantially increase premiums, you would at least have the option of continuing coverage with your current term carrier.

A convertible policy, on the other hand, provides the insured with the option to convert the term policy to a permanent policy at some time in the future. Once again, this may be accomplished without proof of insurability or medical underwriting. Some term carriers will provide both a renewable as well as a convertible policy provisions with their contracts.

Other provisions, known as riders, can be added to certain policies for an additional cost. The waiver of premium rider allows the policy owner to actually stop making premium payments if he or she becomes disabled and is unable to work and earn an income. The accidental death rider would obligate the insurance company to pay out to your beneficiary double or in some cases even triple the stated death benefit if you die in an accident.

A newer rider that is starting to get a lot of attention is the accelerated death benefit. You may be able to receive a portion of your own death benefit while you are alive, in the event you have a major medical condition, such as metastatic cancer, chronic renal failure, or pancreatic cancer, that is expected to lead to death within a short period of time. This rider will provide needed funds immediately to help with medical bills or other support issues during a terminal illness.

Permanent Insurance

Permanent insurance needs are solved through varying types of whole life and universal life policies designed to stay in force throughout one's lifetime. Unlike term insurance where premiums generally increase as the insured gets older, most permanent life insurance premiums remain level. These policies combine the death benefit protection of term insurance with a savings element known as "cash value."

Life insurance cash values grow on a tax-deferred basis, thus creating a supplemental tax-advantaged savings vehicle. Unlike other tax-deferred vehicles such as IRAs, retirement plans, and annuities, life insurance cash values are not subject to the minimum penalty free withdrawal age of 59½. In addition, and of particular interest to physicians, is the fact that in many states, life insurance cash values and the death benefits (assuming there is a named beneficiary) are shielded from creditors, thus creating an effective asset-protection strategy. The accumulated cash values form a reserve that enables the insurer to pay a policy's full death benefit while keeping premiums level. Depending on the specific life insurance company, cash values of permanent life insurance policies may be withdrawn or borrowed over the life of the policy. Cash-value loans or withdrawals can also be used to supplement retirement income or fund college education costs.

The main attribute of whole life insurance is the inherent guarantee that as long as premium payments are paid in a timely manner, the policy will remain in force regardless of any changes in the insured's health.

Universal life insurance policies differ from whole life policies by separating the various components of the policy, such as cash value, mortality costs (the actual cost of the insurance), and other expenses. This allows the insurance company to build a higher level of flexibility into the contract, which in turn provides the policyholder with the ability to make adjustments in response to changing needs and circumstances. This flexibility can include the amount and frequency of future premium payments, as well as the ability to reduce the amount of the death benefit as one's net worth increases.

Whether it is a traditional whole life or universal life insurance policy, it is important to understand the variables that affect the growth of your cash value over time. Most permanent insurance cash-value increases are due to the dividend-paying ability of the insurance company (based on the company's earnings and profitability) or through the insurance company's own investment returns expressed as an interest rate percentage (interest rate sensitive insurance). In both cases, insurance companies offer a guaranteed minimum amount, or interest rate percentage, that they will credit to the policy.

With interest-rate sensitive policies, which are the most common type used in universal life, the insurance company invests its cash assets in relatively conservative investment vehicles such as government and high-grade corporate bonds, although it may also diversify into equities and real estate. The results of the investment strategy are passed through to the policyholders via cash-value additions at a specific interest rate.

Variable life insurance, whether it's a whole or universal life policy, actually allows policyholders to have more control over the growth of their cash-value account. Policyholders can allocate a portion of each premium payment to one or more investment sub accounts or separate investment options, based on their specific risk tolerance and long-term growth objective. Deductions for expenses and mortality charges are taken by the insurance company prior to the allocation to the specific sub accounts.

Most variable life policies offer the policyholders a wide range of investment options, including various stock and bond mutual funds. Depending on the specific insurance company, options may include index funds, real estate funds, foreign stock funds, small company, and other types of sector funds. Also included may be a fixed account option in which the insurer guarantees a fixed rate of return.

Keep in mind that with most cash-value life insurance policies, there may be substantial surrender charges associated with canceling or terminating the policy. These charges are generally highest in the early years of a policy and usually decline over time, typically after 7–15 years, depending on the specific insurance company. If your needs have changed since you purchased the policy, you do have options other than just surrendering the policy. Permanent insurance options may also include the ability to suspend premium payments, while at the same time, maintain some level of coverage on a reduced basis.

Based on the amount of cash value within the policy, life insurance illustrations can be prepared to determine the feasibility of actually lowering the face amount of the death benefit, thus lowering the mortality cost within the contract. This is accomplished by determining the amount of reduced benefit that can be supported by the current level of cash values. In this manner, you may still be able to take a partial withdrawal or loan against the policy now or in the future, but avoid full surrender, thus eliminating any insurance company-imposed surrender charges and any potential income tax liability.

If the desire is not to reduce the amount of the death benefit, then another option to explore is the feasibility of converting the permanent policy to a paid-up term insurance policy. An analysis will determine how long the term coverage will remain in force, based on the mortality cost of the coverage. If this strategy is implemented, the cash value is used to pay for the paid-up term coverage, thus eliminating any ability to access cash values in the future.

You can, however, access cash values without terminating a policy via cash-value withdrawals or through loans. Policy cash-value loans allow the policyholder to borrow a portion of their cash-value account. The rate charged by the insurance company is typically lower than current market loan rates. The loan may not have to be repaid, but if there is an outstanding policy loan, the company will reduce the death benefit if the insured dies before the loan is repaid.

LONG-TERM CARE INSURANCE

Shopping for long-term care insurance policies is similar to comparing different long-term disability policies. As with disability coverage, the benefits covered as well as the dollar limitations dictate the pricing of the policy. Begin by determining what levels of care you would like to insure against.

One factor to consider is housing. The aging of America has forced many senior citizens and their families to explore the myriad housing options available today. Housing choices for the elderly include independent living, assisted living, nursing homes, continuing care communities, and staying at home.

Independent living housing is an attractive option for active seniors who can take care of themselves and prefer a social versus medical setting. The facility typically can accommodate a broad range of lifestyles and often includes activities and transportation to shopping and other outside events. Many also have dining rooms that serve daily meals, though most independent living facilities include a full kitchen within the resident's apartment or living unit.

Residents can enjoy daily activities without worrying about typical maintenance and repairs of their homes. If ongoing medical care becomes a need, options include hiring a private aide (at the residents own cost) or moving to an assisted living or nursing home facility.

Assisted living facilities essentially are communities designed for seniors who have some level of difficulty living and managing on their own. They provide a moderate level of personal care, including assistance with bathing and administering medications. Individual living units, which are usually rented on a monthly basis, are typically small, with limited kitchens or no no cooking facilities at all. Additional care may be available to residents at an additional cost. Typically, assisted living facilities are less expensive but more comfortable than nursing homes.

Nursing homes offer a much more intense level of medical care and attention, usually under the supervision of a medical doctor. With so many other elderly care options available today, nursing homes have become geared toward dementia patients, limited rehabilitation stays, or patients near the end of their lives. Nursing homes can provide almost hospital-quality medical care for chronic illnesses, but at a lower cost. As opposed to monthly fees, nursing homes charge on a daily basis. Private rooms may be difficult to find and cost-prohibitive.

Continuing care communities, also known as life care communities, attempt to provide facilities for all stages of aging within the same housing complex, and include independent and assisted living, as well as nursing and rehabilitative care. Costs include substantial entry fees plus monthly payments. The major advantage here is the ease of movement between levels of care as the resident's condition changes. From a social standpoint, seniors may still maintain contact with friends as they move within the community.

Staying at home, with its familiar surroundings and proximity to friends and neighbors, remains the top choice for many seniors. By avoiding change, seniors can maintain an important sense of independence. Hired care can be tailored to specific situations, and the aides provide a more personal one-on-one care environment. The difficulty comes with transportation issues relative to shopping and other errands, as well as the relatively high level of turnover of home health aides.

Again, the benefits covered as well as the dollar limitations dictate the pricing of the policy. When determining what levels of care you would like to insure against consider the definitions within the policies, which may include the following:

1. *Skilled Care:* Physician-ordered daily nursing and possibly rehabilitation care under the supervision of licensed skilled registered nurses and other skilled medical personnel.

2. *Intermediate Care:* Same skilled personnel as above, except care is required only occasionally, not daily.

3. *Custodial Care:* Based on doctor's orders, assistance may be covered within the policy for help with daily activities such as bathing, eating, dressing, mobility issues, etc. The assistance generally does not need to be provided by skilled medical personnel.

Certain policies will also cover home health care coverage, either as part of the policy or as an added-on rider. Other determinants of premium pricing include: maximum allowable daily dollar limitations, inflation protection, guaranteed renewability, and a waiver of premium based on a specified number of days spent in a nursing home.

The funding of long-term care expenses, which include the cost of a nursing home as well as other care expenses, can come from personal savings and investments, retirement plan benefits, or from long-term care insurance. One of the biggest misconceptions comes from the belief that Medicare will provide these benefits. Medicare does not provide coverage for nursing homes, though Medicaid may if all conditions are met.

INDIVIDUAL RETIREMENT ACCOUNTS

A final step prior to leaving a practice is to ensure that if you have a retirement plan, you take the necessary steps to avoid taxation and penalties as the assets leave the previous employer's plan. This is typically accomplished through the use of an IRA (Individual Retirement Account) rollover. The rules for moving money from retirement accounts are the same as if you had an IRA that you wanted to move to another IRA account. Alternatively, if the new practice allows the rollover from the previous employer's plan, you will need to determine if the plan offers you the best opportunity for growth.

If you find you are between jobs and you need cash, the IRA rollover can help with those financial needs during this time. If you withdraw funds from an IRA but redeposit the money back into an IRA within 60 days, there are no current income tax ramifications. When all of the requirements are met, IRA rollovers are tax-free and exempt from the usual 10% penalty on early withdrawals before age 59½.

However, it is important to keep in mind several potential pitfalls with IRA-to-IRA rollovers:

1. *Missing the 60-day rollover period.* The rollover must be completed within 60 days after the date a distribution is made from the old IRA. For years, the IRS ruled the 60-day requirement could not be waived, even when the

delay was not the taxpayer's fault. Recently, the IRS indicated that it's more willing to grant an exception or waiver under extenuating circumstances, but it is still best to play it safe and stay within the 60-day rollover period.

2. *Failure to roll over the same assets that were distributed.* To qualify for a tax-free rollover, the cash or other assets withdrawn from the old IRA must be transferred within 60 days. You are not allowed to substitute other property. For example, in a recent tax court case, an individual withdrew cash from his IRA and used the money to invest in common stocks. He then transferred the stocks to a new IRA within the required 60-day rollover period. The tax court ruled that the transfer was taxable, since there was a change in the distributed assets.

3. *Rolling over to the wrong IRA.* The tax-advantaged rollover is valid only if you make a timely rollover to an IRA that you personally own. If you mistakenly transfer the rollover funds to your spouse's IRA or some other account, the transfer is fully taxable.

4. *Initiating more than one rollover during the year.* You are allowed to roll over funds from one IRA to another IRA only once a year. The one-year period begins on the date you receive the distribution, not the date on which you roll over the funds into the IRA. The one-year rollover rule applies separately to each IRA that you own.

5. *Rolling over a mandatory distribution.* The law requires you to begin minimum distributions from an IRA by April 1 of the year following the year in which you reach age 70½. You cannot avoid the minimum distribution rule by rolling over the distribution to another IRA. Mandatory distributions may be avoided if the retirement plan assets are not held within an IRA, but are kept within the plan, and you have not yet retired. This exception, however, is not available for distributions made within an IRA.

6. *Rolling over IRA assets to a Roth IRA.* In general, the rollover from a regular IRA to a Roth IRA is completely taxable, but the funds will be able to be withdrawn tax-free after the mandatory five-year holding period.

Regardless if you roll over the funds to the new plan or to an IRA, be certain to complete proper beneficiary designations.

With most physicians' IRA generally representing their largest financial asset, it makes sense to everything possible to avoid retirement account mistakes. While many institutions provide custody services for IRA assets, the onus is on the IRA owner to make the most of the rules, while avoiding the most common traps both in the law and in those created by custodians.

The most common mistake physicians make with IRAs relates to the designation of beneficiary. As each IRA is established, whether at a bank, brokerage firm, trust company, or mutual fund, you are required to complete a beneficiary designation form. What makes this form so critical is that it, not your will or trust, will determine who will inherit this valuable asset. Individuals who aren't quite sure frequently name their estate as their beneficiary. Consequently, at the time of their death, their entire IRA will need to be fully distributed over five years. If distributions have already begun, then the payouts will continue based on the initial projected life expectancy of the deceased.

Typically, IRA owners name a spouse as beneficiary while not naming or giving very little consideration to who the contingent beneficiary should be. Based on current and updated tax law, there are now greater advantages to naming children or grandchildren. If your spouse predeceases you, or survives you but is financially comfortable enough not to need the distributions from the IRA, the children or grandchildren will be able to stretch out the distributions over their own life expectancies, thus creating a longer period of tax-deferred accumulation.

In the event one of the named children dies prior to the IRA owner, the deceased child's portion of the inheritance goes to the other living children, as opposed to the deceased child's family. This may be your objective. If on the other hand, your desire is to have that child's portion pass through to his or her heirs, be sure to add the line: "to my descendants per stirpes." This specific legal jargon will ensure that if the beneficiary child dies, his or her descendants get the full share.

Also keep in mind that if for any reason the IRA custodian form doesn't allow for much beneficiary designation flexibility, they will often allow you to submit an attachment that better clarifies your wishes.

PROFESSIONAL GUIDANCE

As you can see, physicians face many financial issues early in their career. Working with a financial advisor can certainly make this process more efficient. The relationship with one's financial advisor is a true partnership where both parties are working toward a common goal: your financial stability and financial independence. A financial advisor may help manage your insurance programs and investments, perform portfolio evaluations, and serve as an educator to ensure a greater understanding of the financial planning environment.

In addition to registered investment advisors, there are a number of other financial-based professionals who may be in a position to assist you with many financial planning areas. The following list of professionals, as well as their industry-focused professional designations, and educational requirements, should serve as a guide in your search for advice:

- *Certified Financial Planner (CFP®)*. The Certified Financial Planner Board of Standards is a regulatory organization for financial planners that awards the CFP® designation to individuals who meet its requirements. The curriculum covers insurance, income taxation, retirement planning, investments, and estate planning. In addition to self-study programs, classroom instruction is offered at colleges and universities across the country.
- *Chartered Life Underwriter (CLU)*. The CLU self-study curriculum includes 10 courses: 8 required and 2 electives. Three years of business experience and client service in the financial field are prerequisites for the course.
- *Chartered Financial Consultant (CHFC)*. The CHFC self-study program includes 10 courses: 9 required and 1 elective. Three years of business experience and client service in the financial field are required.

As is the case with all professional designations, having one does not necessarily mean you are good at what you do. Word of mouth through referrals made by friends and colleagues is an excellent way to meet potential advisors. Even though they may come highly recommended, it is always a good idea to interview a number of advisors to determine compatibility. Only in this manner will you be able to determine who you are most comfortable partnering with in guiding you toward reaching, and ultimately maintaining, true financial independence and long-term security.

SUMMARY

Most beginning physicians are so eager to begin the practice of medicine that they overlook such important issues as disability insurance, life insurance, and retirement planning. Prudent doctors will begin practice with the security that they will be taken care of if disabled, that their family will be properly cared for in the event of death, and that ample funds are going to available when they decide to retire or leave the medical profession. This requires planning, and the best time to start the planning process is the day you start your practice. Waiting to make these plans can be a costly and in some cases irreparable mistake.

CHAPTER 7

Renewing Yourself: The Key Role of Work–Life Balance

Peter S. Moskowitz, MD

STRESS AND PROFESSIONAL BURNOUT are becoming major concerns for physicians nationwide. Although the problem has long been recognized as one of the hazards of the practice of medicine, solutions are not always readily at hand. I cannot over-emphasize the importance of work-life balance as the best insulator against professional burnout.

MEET DR. W.

Dr. W., age 47, sought career-coaching services to help him with his "unmanageable" life. As a hospital-based specialist in private practice, he found the increasing pressures in his professional practice had begun to negatively affect his private life. He was working 11-hour days regularly, every third weekend and every fifth weekday on-call, averaging 70 hours of work and call per week.

In addition, Dr. W. chaired two important hospital committees, served as clinical director of his hospital department, and maintained a teaching appointment at the nearby medical school on his one afternoon off each week. He described himself as "bored" and frequently loses his temper with patients, nurses, and fellow physicians.

He was weeks behind in personal correspondence and email, hadn't taken a vacation in 10 months, and was having trouble sleeping soundly. At home, his wife and children had begun complaining that he seemed withdrawn and uninterested in their lives. "All I want to do when I get home is zone-out in front of the TV," he explained. "I know I can't go on like this much longer. The money is good, but I'm worried I will lose my health, my sanity, my family, or all of them. I just don't know what to do."

Dr. W. had considered leaving medicine entirely—it was the only solution he could think of. "I guess I'm burned out."

DEFINING THE PROBLEM

The story of Dr. W. is not unusual in my physician coaching practice. Although the time demands on physicians have always been great, the impact of managed care has further increased these demands. Increased use of healthcare services, the expanding numbers of the newly insured, shorter contact time with patients, the impact of electronic medical record systems, loss of autonomy in scheduling their time, and decreasing reimbursement for physician services are all increasing physician stress.

Doctors are working more and often for less money these days. Hospital certification and recertification processes demand more committee time and paperwork from physicians. Preparing for recertification examinations for maintenance of specialty certification eats into their free time on evenings and weekends. There is pressure to move patients through diagnostic evaluations and treatment more rapidly. Clinical decision making is frequently modified by or directed entirely by third-party payers. Physicians' RVU output is frequently monitored by management and used to determine salary raises and bonuses.

In a nutshell, physicians believe they have lost control of the practice of medicine. They often are angry and resentful. Too many have poor stress-coping tools. These conditions are a set up for professional burnout.

THE FUNDAMENTALS OF SELF-RENEWAL

Self-renewal is the general process by which individuals sustain their personal and career health. For 21st-century physicians to be effective, efficient, and healthy, they must be knowledgeable about career-renewal techniques. Outlined here are seven strategies for sustaining self-renewal.

1. Institute personal wellness.

Self-care is a problem for many physicians. We have been trained to take care of our patients first and foremost. Too often that comes at the expense of poor attention to ourselves, to our own health, and to our emotional needs. Here are some strategies for promoting good health and wellness.

- Eat a healthy diet and don't skip meals.
- Exercise aerobically for at least 30 minutes, at least three days a week.
- Sleep at least seven hours every night, preferably eight.
- Have a personal physician (not yourself) and have an annual physical examination.
- Have a personal plan for preventative medicine.
- Have fun daily.

2. Manage your stress effectively and use healthy coping strategies.

In my experience, while physicians use many strategies to manage their stress, some of the strategies are less effective and less healthy than others. Healthy and effective coping strategies include aerobic exercise, prayer, meditation, yoga, travel, connecting to loved ones, and using a support network of friends and colleagues. The less-effective, unhealthy coping strategies include using drugs/alcohol, getting angry and venting, denial, and avoiding difficult situations or people. Doctors who use positive coping skills are happier and experience less burnout.

3. Know and re-assess your purpose and values annually.

Effective professionals have a clear sense of the purpose of their lives and careers. Your purpose serves as your compass in life and helps you set limits and boundaries. Your personal values define what is most important to you regarding ethical questions and the use of your vital resources of time and money. Because our lives are dynamic, we should re-evaluate our personal purpose and our values every year or two.

4. Balance your life.

Work-life balance is the most effective single strategy to protect healthcare professionals from burnout. Work-life balance constitutes a series of six domains, defined and discussed in much greater detail below.

5. Develop a support network and a supportive community.

No man is an island. The hectic lifestyle and the training of physicians often result in doctors having few intimate friends and being reluctant to confide their concerns, weaknesses, and mistakes to others. Lonely and socially isolated, most physicians tend to select other doctors as friends—doctors whose values and thinking parallel theirs. Consequently, they get no objective feedback from people whose value systems and outlooks are different (and healthier) than their own.

To promote resilience and health, physicians should seek out and use a reliable support network. This network may include trusted friends, family members, professional associates, mental health professionals, career/life coaches, and clergy. In addition, physicians benefit from associating with communities of people who share their hobbies, interests, or values. Such communities can provide friendship, advice, and consolation in challenging times.

6. Utilize values-based time and money management.

Our vital resources of time and money, if not managed effectively, can become sources of great stress. Physicians whose lives are out of balance often "overspend" both their time and their money. The solution is to clarify one's personal values concerning time and money, write them down, and re-read them when faced with important decisions about how to spend those resources.

7. Build good communication skills.

The two most important communication skills an effective physician needs are the ability to do reflective listening and to explain complex clinical matters in simple, easy-to-understand language.

Reflective listening means listening to someone, then repeating back to them the exact details of what they said to you. Too often the busy physician starts thinking about how he or she is going to respond to a patient or colleague before the patient or colleague has even finished talking. Reflective listening is a powerful way to build trust and confidence between two people, improve patient satisfaction, and demonstrate that you are truly paying attention. Anyone can master reflective listening with a little practice.

Learning to speak in understandable, layman's terms is also a skill that can be acquired through practice. In all conversations with patients and their families, physicians should strive to describe diagnoses, procedures, and discussions of prognosis with evidence-based conclusions using language that people with little education in science can understand.

LIFESTYLE BALANCE: THE MOST EFFECTIVE RENEWAL TOOL

Lifestyle balance can insulate healthcare professionals against burnout and restore personal and professional resilience. Until recently, the principles and practice of lifestyle balance were not part of the curriculum of our medical schools, and in many medical schools still are not. The culture of American medicine generally has not been sympathetic to physicians wanting to take better care of themselves or to ask for help. The grueling hours of medical training make sustaining lifestyle balance particularly difficult. Studies come first. Patients always come first. As a direct result, medical students, residents, fellows, and practicing physicians typically do not have lifestyle balance.

Many physicians do not have a clear vision of what balance entails or how to acquire it, even if the value of balance is apparent to them. Most have lived their entire professional lives out of balance, believing it is the price they must pay to follow their calling to clinical medicine.

Defining Lifestyle Balance

Any meaningful discussion of lifestyle balance must first define the term and its parameters. The domains of balance for purposes of this discussion include physical balance, emotional balance, spiritual balance, relationship balance, community balance, and work/career balance.

Physical Balance refers to wellness, body conditioning, cardiovascular and musculoskeletal conditioning, strength, endurance, body flexibility, and resistance to disease. People who are physically balanced are in good physical health and condition and have abundant energy.

Emotional Balance refers to a state of calmness, feeling centered, resilient. People who are emotionally balanced are able to accept positive and negative input without excessive mood swings, are relaxed and confident. They have emotional intelligence—that is to say, they are aware of, accept, and manage their own feelings.

Spiritual Balance refers to a state of connectedness to self, to a community, to a power beyond oneself. When spiritually balanced, one feels a part of a greater whole, as if one belongs where one is, and is predominantly hopeful rather than fearful.

Relationship Balance refers to a state in which one is able to receive in a relationship to others to a similar degree that one gives to that relationship; feeling connected to others; being able to comfortably state one's needs, wants, and sense of reality to others without fear of being adversely judged or rejected.

Community Balance refers to having a relationship to some community of people in which what one gives of oneself to that community is balanced by what one receives back from it. This creates energy, gratitude, and selflessness.

Work/Career Balance refers to an elusive sense of giving to work/career enough to be valued as a worker, to succeed, advance, and be challenged, yet without losing one's sense of self or individual values in the process. This is a highly individual domain, unique to each individual and each work setting. It is subject to change over time and within any given job.

Establishing Lifestyle Balance

The most difficult task for those who seek lifestyle balance is recognizing their own lack of balance. Most healthcare professionals, especially physicians early in their training, deny their emotions and their physical and emotional needs as a means of surviving. Physicians-in-training are taught directly and indirectly to "work until the work is done," to "be tough" emotionally and physically, not to feel excessive sympathy, sadness, or emotional pain lest they be ineffective in times of emergency or crisis. Eventually many physicians shut down access to their own emotions so effectively that they are unable to be intimate or real with themselves or with others. Not until they perceive the pain of their own isolation and loneliness as a problem will most physicians seek help in achieving balance.

Working 70-hour weeks, working months on end without a weekend away or a vacation, having no sense of fun in their lives, not taking good physical or spiritual care of themselves—these are all common characteristics of healers. They perceive and problem solve around the needs of others, but not themselves. If not recognized and addressed, dysfunction and crisis eventually intervene in their lives and relationships.

The equation to reach lifestyle balance is unique to each individual. It is a dynamic equation that changes over time, yet consistently will lead to a greater sense of well-being. Lifestyle balance is the most potent insulator from stress and burnout for the physician and other healthcare professionals.

To acquire better balance, the physician must learn to assess his or her needs in all the domains of balance on a daily basis. This self-awareness must come from a daily practice of listening to the inner voice through prayer, meditation, journaling, or quiet time alone. Establishing such time "just to be" is one of the most difficult tasks for busy physicians. They have been trained to consider such time as wasted, nonproductive. Physicians' self-esteem depends largely on productivity and achievement.

As their lives become more balanced, physicians begin to value their time alone. They become happy with what they have and, if not, are proactive in changing those things they can control in order to get what they want. Maintaining balance also requires that physicians assess their personal values and integrate those values into their daily lives and their time-management strategies.

An integral progression toward work–life balance relates to how physicians spend their time. Balance does not mean finding a way to rush from one domain to the next throughout the day, hoping to spend a bit of time in each. Rather, it requires a *synthesis* or *integration* of values, career, and private life so as to reinforce their values and spend as much time each day satisfying their domain requirements simultaneously. This may require major career reengineering as well as classic time-management training.

Once the concept of balance is established and under conscious scrutiny, the consequences of lifestyle *imbalance* may become more apparent through counseling, journaling, and/or meditation practice. Physicians may recognize recurrent behaviors and consequences that adversely affect their career, personal, or family life and provide meaningful material to facilitate lifestyle change.

The Personal Craziness Index, developed by Patrick Carnes, is useful for daily self-monitoring of lifestyle balance. Originally created to facilitate healthy lifestyle choices for people in addiction recovery, it is also useful for physicians, whose obsessive-compulsive personality may respond well to this approach for monitoring balance.

THE SPECIAL CASE: MEDICAL STUDENTS, INTERNS, RESIDENTS, AND FELLOWS

Even though medical students and physician trainees understand and value the concept of living a balanced life, their academic and training environments make that objective supremely challenging for several reasons:

1. Their academic demands can be overwhelming at times.
2. Because of their limited life experience, their innate competitiveness, and the familiarity of living life in a "full-court-press" mode, they may not have developed good stress management tools.
3. Medical schools and training institutions do not commonly address students' and trainees' career planning and wellness needs, leaving young physicians without the kind of support they really need.
4. Students and trainees who have no regular life partner have no one but themselves to provide for their own basic needs and services. They must manage to squeeze those activities in between all of the other demands placed upon them.
5. Individual performance rewards in medical school as well as in training are based on success in "doing" rather than on "being." As a result, students and trainees may see no inherent value in working hard at self-care and balancing.
6. Although faculty and attending physicians are role models for students and trainees, many live their own lives and careers out of balance, sending the wrong message to their charges.

The strategies for balancing life and work that students and trainees find successful are similar, if not identical to those used by practicing physicians. However, the unique environment of medical school and house officer training programs suggests some different approaches. The strategies below have proven useful in my work with students and trainees. The more that can be successfully incorporated into daily life, the better the outcome.

1. Use an electronic calendar on your smartphone to manage classes, appointments, call schedules, and personal activities. It helps to prevent lapses of memory when you are stressed and fatigued.
2. Plan your seven-day weekly schedule on Sundays and enter the activities into your electronic calendar.

3. Put yourself on your schedule; provide time for exercise, fun, and connection to others.
4. Find time for aerobic exercise at least three days a week, for at least 30 minutes.
5. Eat nutritious food, eat meals regularly, and never skip meals no matter how busy you are.
6. To the extent possible, avoid the mood-altering effects of excessive sugar and caffeine.
7. Stay connected with family, friends, and loved ones. Electronic communication using smartphones, social media, Skype, or FaceTime facilitate such contact.
8. Cultivate relationships with cohorts and adults inside and outside medicine who will support you in difficult times.
9. Seek out and meet regularly with faculty and/or attending physician mentors.
10. Schedule 5–10 minutes of fun of any kind on a daily basis, and more on free weekends, days off clinical service, and vacations.
11. Identify and make use of spiritual tools, which can include reading spiritual sources, meditating, praying, spending quiet time alone, being out in nature, and participating in spiritual communities of your choice.
12. To the extent possible, regulate your bedtime and awakening time, and aim for at least seven hours of sleep when not on call or working in hospitals.
13. Maintain interests and hobbies outside of medicine.

EFFECTIVE STRATEGIES FOR LIFESTYLE BALANCE

Strategies for achieving work–life balance must be flexible, challenging, and address all six of the life balance domains. While not all-inclusive, the techniques and strategies below have proven valuable. They are listed by domain.

PHYSICAL BALANCE

1. Institute and maintain a physician-directed wellness program to include at least 30 minutes of aerobic exercise at least three days per week and a low-fat, high-fiber diet to promote healthy body weight and blood lipid profile.
2. Obtain a physician-generated assessment (not a self-assessment) of physical health annually.
3. Tap into previous sports passions and physical skills to sustain and energize the exercise program. Schedule these programs—preferably before the start of the workday.
4. Explore hidden desires and take risks. Both are challenges for personal growth. They also support self-esteem and self-confidence while making positive lifestyle changes.

EMOTIONAL BALANCE

1. Develop a daily program for self-awareness. Techniques might include any or all of the following: journaling, dream analysis, prayer, mindfulness meditation, and quiet time alone.
2. Think in terms of acceptance and letting go of all that is beyond your control. The Serenity Prayer is a starting point.
3. Use mindfulness training to stay in the moment, letting go of what happened yesterday and not worrying about what may happen tomorrow.
4. Develop a support network. This may include a same-sex professional colleague, psychotherapist, career/life coach, men's/women's group, spiritual discussion group, hobby group. Having support from others outside of your immediate family is healthy and reduces the emotional burden on your spouse, significant other, and other family members.
5. Utilize Carnes' Personal Craziness Index.

SPIRITUAL BALANCE

1. Be clear about the difference between *spiritual* and *religious*.
2. Participate in activities that you find to be spiritually uplifting at least weekly.
3. Seek a spiritual advisor (clergy, friend, mentor) who can help you sustain and grow your spiritual practice and knowledge.
4. Make a list of spiritual activities and decide which ones appeal to you. Make a commitment to yourself to begin a program of spiritual practice.
5. Use mindfulness training to stay in the moment.
6. Learn to enjoy spontaneous fun, especially with spouse, partner, and children. Take clues from your favorite childhood activities and/or those of your children. You may need to schedule "spontaneous fun" at first.
7. Learn to listen to and act upon your own inner voice. This skill can best be developed in conjunction with self-awareness practice(s) already established.
8. Consider that the practice of self-care of the body is a spiritual practice.
9. Learn to accept emotional pain and fear as teachers, as a normal part of living. Spiritual growth occurs when we learn to confront pain and fear, not run away from them.

RELATIONSHIP BALANCE

1. Develop a relationship with yourself. This can be accomplished through a self- awareness program, spiritual practice, and time alone.
2. Set annual life goals and reassess progress annually, with the support and feedback of others.

3. Do an annual assessment of "give and take" in all of your major relationships. This helps you to visualize whether you are predominantly a giver or a taker. Revise these roles when appropriate.

4. Understand and practice the principle of reflective listening—seeking to understand rather than to respond when conversing with others.

WORK/CAREER BALANCE

1. Understand the fundamentals of the Cycle of Renewal.
2. Understand that work/career rewards are not linear in relation to effort.
3. Determine your financial goals and integrate them with your career values. Use a certified financial planner if needed.
4. Learn to take risks at work and accept new challenges as a way to sustain career resilience.
5. Accept responsibility for what you do or do not accomplish at work. We create our own futures.
6. Use medicine as a platform to meet your personal and professional needs in case your current career is no longer satisfactory.
7. Secure the services of a professional coach to help you sustain balance, personal growth, and commitment. Balance in other domains often helps compensate for unhappiness at work.
8. Join or start a physicians' support group.
9. Attend physician wellness programs.
10. Be clear about your passions regarding work and how to pursue them. If conflicts develop in your current job, devise a long-term strategy for transition. Remember that such transitions typically take several years.
11. When you are in career transition, find ways to network with other physicians in transition.

PITFALLS TO ACHIEVING BALANCE

Achieving lifestyle balance is difficult work for even the most committed physicians. Living life in balance requires a paradigm shift that most successful healthcare professionals are not prepared for, nor can they sustain readily by themselves. Success requires a thorough education, an unwavering commitment to change, and a strong support network.

Physicians who fail in their attempt to achieve long-term life balance typically do so by reverting to old behaviors that are more comfortable and easy, especially in times of increasing stress or crisis. The following is a list of some of the reasons physicians fail in their efforts to obtain consistent life balance.

1. Perfectionism

Physicians' perfectionism may provide a disincentive to change by means of procrastination. Afraid they may not do things perfectly, they instead obsess and do nothing. We must see change as a process—one that requires only progress, not perfection.

2. Isolationism

"I can handle this myself" is the battle cry of physicians. If we fail to establish a network for support, there is also no accountability, despite good intentions, to follow through on our commitments to change. For this reason, physicians usually need a good career coach, therapist, or mentor to sustain success in achieving balance in life.

3. Over-commitment

Physicians are typically overly responsible and conscientious. While these attributes generally serve us well, we have a hard time saying no, and easily become overcommitted. While this strategy supports ego to some extent, it distracts from self-esteem to the point that we are often unable to fulfill all of our self-expectations. As a result, it is hard for busy physicians to focus and simplify. We resist taking things "off our plate."

4. Preexisting Addictions

Some physicians adapt to the pain of their own self-denial, stress, the tragedy in their patient's lives, and/or the pain in their own lives in unhealthy ways. Over time, such self-medication of our feelings may become habitual forms of escape. The result is alcohol and/or drug abuse, self-administration of prescription medications, compulsive overeating, compulsive gambling, sexual compulsivity, and work addiction. Some of us become addicted to the urgency in our lives, creating an adrenaline rush by living constantly in crisis to sustain this feeling of intensity.

Help for all such physicians must encompass psychotherapy, education, and 12-step recovery when appropriate. Practice interventions may become necessary to avoid professional and/or legal consequences.

5. Financial Overextension

Although American physicians are among the most highly compensated in the world, we receive little to no education in financial planning during medical school and postgraduate training. And, because we are trusting of others and overcommitted at work, we are easy prey for unscrupulous investment schemes, make poorly informed financial decisions, and often take unwarranted financial risks.

For some, delayed gratification during long years of education and training is followed by self-indulgence once in practice, lifestyles that are hard to sustain in these times of cost containment, managed resource allocation, and downsizing. Today, these factors are combining to create financial fears unknown heretofore among physicians.

Physicians find themselves trapped in their careers, perhaps wanting to slow down and cut back, but finding it impossible without abandoning long-held financial objectives (e.g., financing college education for their children, early retirement) or downsizing their current lifestyle, or both. These financial fears alone prevent many physicians from making the career changes necessary to achieve the life balance they so desire.

Extensive financial planning with our spouses/partners is often helpful. Both partners in the relationship must realistically reassess their short- and long-term financial goals for themselves as individuals and as a couple. Where they disagree, or goals diverge, they must reach difficult compromises. This often requires help from a couples therapist, in addition to a skilled certified financial planner.

Financial over-commitment is the most common and the most difficult hurdle for physicians to overcome in achieving sustainable life balance.

FOLLOWING UP WITH DR. W.

Dr. W has remained in a lifestyle coaching relationship for over a year, meeting for an hour once a week. Initial work focused on reassessing his purpose and identifying his personal and professional values. Time management processes revealed a desire for more renewal time, more family and spouse time, and less time at work.

Dr. W. decided to accomplish these goals by resigning from his hospital committee work, cutting back his practice load by 20%, and recommitting to his medical school teaching role, which energized him. He began a wellness program, lost 20 pounds, and started playing tennis twice a week with several non-physician friends. He learned to schedule time for his two children weekly and a "date" with his wife each weekend when not on call.

He started taking two- to three-day vacations each quarter and longer vacations twice a year. He enriched his spiritual program by joining his church choir. He and his wife slowly revised their financial plan, and Mrs. W. decided to go back to work part time as a nurse to help manage the income reduction from Dr. W's practice. She is enjoying the professional challenge. Both Dr. W. and Mrs. W. are feeling energized, more committed to their marriage, and are once again optimistic about their future in medicine.

SUMMARY

Life balance is the single most powerful insulator against professional burnout. Effective professional career counseling or coaching strategies must educate physicians about the nature of and the major domains of life balance, then seek a commitment from the physician to develop practical daily strategies aimed at establishing balance in all seven domains. While sustaining life balance is a great challenge, the rewards include renewed energy, passion, positive outlook, and renewed commitments to work and personal relationships. Those rewards are well worth the effort.

Resources

Blau J, Harris S, Moskowitz PS and Paprocki R., eds. *Medical Practice Divorce*. Chicago: AMA Press; 2001.

Carnes P. *A Gentle Path Through the Twelve Steps*. Minneapolis, MN: Compcare Publishers;1993.

Clever L. *The Fatigue Prescription. Four Steps to Renewing Tour Energy, Health, and Life*. Berkeley, CA: Cleiss Press; 2010.

Cohn KH, Panasuk, DB, and Holland JC. Workplace Burnout; Identifying Early Signs and Instituting Ongoing Programs to Prevent Disasters. In: Cohn KH, ed. *Better Communication for Better Care: Mastering Physician-Administrator Collaboration*. Chicago: Health Administration Press; 2005.

Covey SR, Merrill AR, and Merrill RR. *First Things First*. New York: Simon and Schuster; 1994.

Drummond D. *Stop Physician Burnout: What to Do When Working Harder Isn't Working*. Collinsville, MS: Heritage Press Publications, LLC; 2014

Dyrbye LN, Shanafelt, TD. Physician burnout. A potential threat to successful health care reform. *JAMA*. 2011 May 18:305(19):2009–10

Dyrbye LN, Varkey P, Boone SL, Satele DV, Sloan JA, and Shanafelt TD. Physician satisfaction and burnout at different career stages. *Mayo Clin Proc*. 2013 Dec;88(12):1358–67.

Eckleberry-Hunt J, Van Dyke A, Lick D, Tucciarone J. Changing the conversation from burnout to wellness: Physician well-being in residency training programs. *J Grad Med Educ*. 2009 Dec:1(2):225–230.

Edelwich J with Brodsky A. *Burn-Out: Stages of Disillusionment in the Helping Professions*. New York: Human Science Press; 1980.

Freudenberger H and Richelson G. (1980). *Burnout: The High Cost of Achievement*. New York: Bantam; 1980.

Gautam M. IronDoc: *Practical Stress Management Tools for Physicians*. Ontario, CN: Book Coach Press; 2004.

Gerber L. *Married to Their Careers: Career and Family Dilemmas in Doctors' Lives*. New York: Tavistock Publications; 1983.

Hudson FM and McLean O. *LifeLaunch: A Passionate Guide to the Rest of Your Life*. Santa Barbara, CA. Hudson Institute Press; 1995.

Jaffe D and Scott C. *From Burnout to Balance: A Workbook for Peak Performance and Staff Renewal.* New York: McGraw-Hill Book Co.;1984.

Kabat-Zinn J. *Wherever You Go, There You Are: Mindfulness Meditation in Everyday Life.* New York: Hyperion; 1994.

Keeton K, Fenner DE, Johnson TR, and Hayward RA. Predictors of physician career satisfaction, work-life balance, and burnout. *Obstet Gynecol.* 2007 Apr;109(4): 949-55. 2007

Linzer M, Levine R, Meltzer D, Poplau S, Warde C, West CP. 10 gold steps to prevent burnout in general internal medicine. *J. Gen Intern Med.* 2014 Jan;29(1):18–20. 2014.

Lipsenthal L. *Finding Balance in a Medical Life.* 2007. San Anselmo, CA: Lee Lipsenthal, MD; 2007.

Moskowitz PS. Beyond substance abuse: Stress, burnout, and depression as causes of physician impairment and disruptive behavior. *J Am Coll Radiol.* 2010 Apr;7(4): 313–4.

Moskowitz PS. Living on borrowed time. *Fam Pract Manag.* 2001 Feb;8(2):66.

Moskowitz PS. Physician renewal: The importance of life balance. *Career Planning and Adult Development Journal.* Spring 1998;14(1):81–92.

Moskowitz PS. Responding to the challenges of stress and burnout. *Diagnostic Imaging.* December 1999;(12):47–49.

Paolini HO, Bertram B, Hamilton T. Antidotes to burnout: Fostering physician resiliency, well-being, and holistic development. *Medscape, Multispecialty.* April 19, 2013.

Pfifferling J-H. Physician well-being. In *Medicine in Transition: Techniques for Coping with Stress and Change* (pp. 21–54). Doctors Resource Service, American Medical Association; July 1984.

Schaufeli WB and Bakker AB. Job demands, job resources, and their relationship with burnout and engagement: A multi-sample study. *J. Organiz. Behav.* March 2004; 25: 293–315.

Shanafelt TD, Boone S, Tan L, Dyrbye LN, Sotile W, Satele D, et al. Burnout and satisfaction with work-life balance among US physicians relative to the general US population. *Arch Intern Med.* 212 Oct 8;172(18):1377–85.

Shrivastava R. How doctors treat doctors may be medicine's secret shame. *The Guardian.* February 6, 2015.

Stecker T. Well-being in an academic environment. *Medical Education.* 2004; 38(5): 465–78.

Wallace, JE, Lemaire, JB, and Ghali, WA. Physician wellness: A missing quality indicator. *Lancet.* 2009; 374(9702): 714–21.

CHAPTER 8

Managing a Practice or Career Transition

Peter S. Moskowitz, MD

THE PAST TWO DECADES BROUGHT profound changes to American medicine. These changes in practice structure, management, and reimbursement models have a significant effect on physicians professionally and personally, as evidenced by widespread career dissatisfaction, increased stress and burnout, increased medical disability claims by doctors, premature retirement, and an increase in the number of physicians changing to non-clinical career options.

Several factors have accelerated this crisis, including changing healthcare drivers, managed care, regionalization of care, mergers and acquisitions of healthcare and physician organizations, the growing loss of physician autonomy, and decreased professional reimbursement.

Physicians and their organizations have responded to these new challenges slowly and without a unified voice. Coupled with the relative paucity of physician coping skills mentioned in Chapter 7, these factors have greatly increased the stress of medical practice. For many, the stresses now exceed the rewards, leading to a significant movement of physicians into new and alternative careers, part-time work, and early retirement.

This chapter is presented with a conscious effort to recognize the scope of the career issues facing physicians and to provide them and their spouses and partners with information, strategies, and tools with which to facilitate planning for career transitions.

CAUSES OF MEDICAL PRACTICE TRANSITIONS

Career Stress and Burnout

The factors that physicians identify as being most responsible for their stress and dissatisfaction include a loss of practice autonomy, increased hours of work, pressure to see more patients in less time, inability to control the work environment, loss of balance between work and private life, and decreasing financial rewards. More recent factors contributing to physician dissatisfaction include the high cost of medical education and education-related debt, the high cost of home ownership in metropolitan areas, and the changing practice and lifestyle expectations of younger physicians.

Physical Illness and Disability

Because they live and work under inordinate stress, physicians are at greater-than-average risk for stress-related illnesses. Disability claims to insurers by physicians are rising alarmingly; this dramatic rise is related proportionately more to emotional disabilities than physical illnesses. Physical illness and disabilities often require modifications of the work environment, creating the need for career transitions.

Emotional and Behavioral Disability

It is a tribute to the medical profession that most doctors function well under the conditions in which they work. However, a steadily increasing number of them are struggling because of emotional and/or behavior problems, such as depression, anxiety disorders, bipolar illness, other psychiatric disorders, and addictions of various types. All these conditions may be exacerbated by stress.

Stress and emotional issues can also lead to behavioral problems. Aggressive, hostile, angry, or other inappropriate behavior in the workplace may result in physician sanctions or other disciplinary consequences that may necessitate a transition.

Burnout, often the end result of chronic stress, has reached epidemic proportions, with as many as 50% of American physicians admitting to at least one symptom of burnout.[1] The emotional turmoil associated with professional burnout may overlap symptoms of psychiatric disorders listed above. The problem of burnout and effective solutions is discussed in Chapter 7.

Skill–Reward Mismatch

This term refers to a physician's discovery, over time, that his or her particular medical skill set is not being adequately recognized or rewarded in the workplace or community. Regardless of the reasons for this discrepancy, the byproduct is resentment. Over time, this resentment increases stress and erodes professional collegiality.

Although purely financial mismatches may be corrected with dynamic marketing, non-financial mismatches such as professional competition within a group are more difficult to rectify. The latter should be a red flag for a physician, indicating the potential need for a practice transition.

Expected vs. Actual Workload Mismatch

Physicians enter practice with certain expectations regarding the intensity of their patient care, night call, and business management responsibilities. In the past decade, managed care has significantly increased the intensity and expectations of patient care contacts per physician work unit, particularly in HMO and multi-specialty clinics.

For many physicians whose professional and personal life balance has been marginal, this change alone has been the single factor that has overwhelmed them, leading to stress, burnout, and the desire for a practice transition.

Personality, Gender, and Generational Conflicts at Work

The American physician has always been considered fiercely independent and self-reliant. Increasingly, these characteristics have become the seeds of interpersonal conflict within physician groups and organizations.

Battles for control and leadership, gender issues (particularly the unequal treatment and/or pay of women physicians), work habits, and professional turf battles are common sources of interpersonal conflict in physician organizations, as are arguments over compensation, workload, and weekend/night call allocation. Struggles between different generations of physicians within a physician organization are becoming standard as Gen-Xers, Gen-Yers, Netsters, and Boomers struggle over differences in perception and attitudes relating to the common issues they share. Any or all of these factors may lead physicians to seek a transition to a more personally satisfying practice setting or a new clinical or non-clinical career.

Relationship Conflicts Outside of the Workplace

Physicians' marriages and relationships fail at a significantly higher rate when compared to the rest of the general population and perhaps even when compared to other professionals. Because of their incomparable work ethic, overwhelming sense of responsibility, and dedication to patients, physicians typically place their clinical practice demands at the top of their list of time priorities, even over family.

Faced with the emotional, physical, and intellectual challenges of a medical career, many physicians return home at the end of the day exhausted unable to sustain or uninterested in emotional intimacy with family, spouse, or companion. Rebuilding the marriage and other family relationships must become a conscious task and a priority. Commitments to improve marriages or relationships lead many physicians to a medical practice transition.

Academic Career Cycle Issues

While physicians in academic practice may experience any and all of the traditional causes of professional practice transition, the nature of academic practice introduces additional factors that may contribute to a decision for a career change. These include difficulties obtaining academic promotion and tenure, skill–reward mismatches relating to clinical care versus research, the politics of academia, and pressures relating to research productivity and research funding.

Junior faculty are expected to excel in clinical care, teaching, and research; the resulting pressures for promotion and the declining numbers of tenured positions often make the environment intense and competitive. Senior faculty may be promoted to positions of departmental management and leadership for which they have little interest or skills.

These pressures lead many faculty to seek better situations at other institutions, modify their academic careers in ways that better suit their own values and skills, or leave academic practice for the perceived greener pastures of private practice or industry.

Changing Skill Sets

As physicians' careers evolve and mature, some clinical or management skills may become stronger or more important, while others may weaken or become less important. Some physicians may find that practice management is a better fit with their interests, skills, and temperament. Others may lose clinical skills owing to changing patient demographics, resulting in less frequent use of certain procedures. Older physicians may elect to stop performing certain high-risk interventions or surgical procedures.

If a physician's desires in this respect are not acceptable to partners, groups, or institutions, the dilemma may not be resolvable by negotiation, creating another reason for a physician to pursue a practice transition.

Retirement and Protirement

When physicians retire from the practice of medicine they go through a natural transition process that is highly variable and individually defined. This transition to retirement living may not go smoothly, particularly if physicians have no well-developed interests outside of medicine or if their financial status or physical health are not stable. Retirement is most successful when physicians have done extensive planning in advance, a process called "protirement."

Protirement, discussed in greater detail in Chapter 13, is most effective when done with the help of a career professional and a certified financial planner. In addition to needing a retirement plan that meets the financial needs of the physician and his or her family, the physician needs a retirement plan that provides ample opportunities for finding personal meaning, a sense of contribution to society, new life challenges, and fun.

NAVIGATING A CAREER TRANSITION

What follows is my approach to understanding and navigating a professional career transition. This approach is equally valid for physicians seeking new careers within or outside of clinical medicine. The theory and strategies are also relevant to physicians who are planning to retire from active practice and seek a life plan that will yield personal meaning and contribution in retirement. Much of the career theory is derived from the work of Frederic Hudson, Ph.D. of the Hudson Institute of Coaching, whose seminal work in this field has been an inspiration for my own coaching career.[2]

When you become aware of your unhappiness, you face three important forks in the road. One fork leads you to keep doing what you have been doing and change nothing. Because change can be frightening, many physicians choose this path until they can no longer hold on.

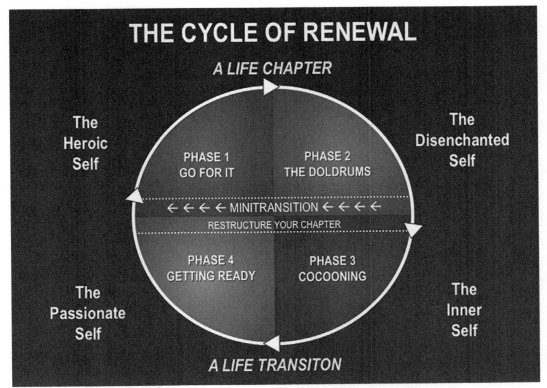

Figure 8-1. Reproduced, with permission, from the Hudson Institute of Coaching.

The second fork in the road leads you to a path crossing the horizontal line dividing the cycle into upper and lower halves. (See Figure 8-1, previous page.) This path will lead you back to Phase 1, Go For It.

You know you will be happy and regain your career passion in Go For It. This path is called a mini-transition. The mini-transition typically takes fewer than six months and does not require a change in location or field of practice. It does, however, require that you acquire new learning and/or a new clinical skill(s). The new skill(s) and learning enable you to attract more patients or new kinds of patients and increase the bottom line in your practice niche. You quickly find yourself back in Phase 1, Go For It! Mini-transitions are popular because they are relatively short in duration and cause much less disruption to the life of a physician and his or her loved ones.

The third path is to scramble out of the doldrums, remain on the perimeter of the career cycle path, and move into Phase 3, into Phase 4, and finally back once more into Phase 1. This third option is called a full-career transition.

THE THREE STAGES OF CAREER TRANSITION

The practical aspects of making a medical career transition can be divided into three stages: Waking Up, Taking Stock, and Taking the Leap of Faith. Note that this process is the same whether the physician is anticipating a transition out of full-time practice, planning a transition to a new full-time or part-time non-medical career, or simply anticipating a transition to retirement.

1. Waking Up

There may come a time when you realize you are unhappy enough to want or need a career change. That's the time to do a brutally honest assessment of what has worked in the job and career and what has not; what is fun and what you hate. Then, determine what is reasonably under your control.

Let go of what is not working or what you hate and hold on to what is working and enjoyable. This is an imperfect and impractical task that will yield temporary relief and provide some clarity. The Serenity Prayer comes to mind: Grant me the serenity to accept the things I cannot change, power to change the things I can, and wisdom to know the difference."

Expect to experience some powerful emotions in this first stage. Early in the transition you may feel out of synch and strangely detached or lost. You will begin to question your entire professional role as a physician and your relationships with other professionals in your field. William Bridges has described this stage as a time of disengagement, dis-identification, disenchantment, and disorientation.[3]

You also may feel energized to be turning over a new leaf, leaving a frustrating position, or starting something new. You may feel anxious and insecure about entering the unknown, about taking new risks. You may feel sad about leaving old friends and comfortable ways.

All of these emotions may be confusing for someone who has always been centered and self-confident. Realize that these emotions and experiences are common to all people in transition. Allow yourself to feel these feelings, recognize and name them. Talk about them with trusted friends and allies, coaches, mentors, therapists, and spouses/partners. Write about them in your journal. Pray and meditate about them in private. Unprocessed feelings may become roadblocks to success in the upcoming transition.

In some ways, when you give up a familiar job, money, prestige, you will go through a grieving process. Kubler-Ross identifies the stages of grieving[4] as denial, anger, bargaining, sadness, and finally acceptance. These stages are not always experienced in this exact sequence, but completing the grieving process requires you to experience all of these feelings, process them, and pass through them to the next chapter of your life.

Processing these feelings can best be done with a professional career coach, mentor, or therapist. Once you establish a plan for the next chapter and begin moving toward that vision for yourself, the uncomfortable feelings of the grief process will pass.

In this first stage of transition it is also important to acknowledge and celebrate what has worked. Plan a formal celebration to remember the good things and the people who have helped make this job and your career a success. Endeavor to leave former jobs and colleagues with a positive memory. Acknowledge their contributions. Do your best not to burn bridges.

2. Taking Stock

During the second stage of career transition, you begin to move out of the Doldrums and into the phase of Cocooning. At this stage, you need to answer a number of important questions before the transition can move forward. Some of the questions are practical and relate to basic resources; others are more elusive questions that probe the very depths of your own self-understanding. These questions include:

1. What financial resources do I have available to assist me in transition? Are they enough? Will these resources support a 3–6 month leave without pay?
2. If my financial resources aren't adequate for an extended time without pay, how much time can I comfortably take to work through my transition

while still working? Do I need to work full time or can I reduce my clinical work to part time?

3. What professional resources (e.g., career coach, therapist, mentor, accountant, financial planner, insurance agent) am I willing and able to make use of?

4. What non-professional sources of support can I make use of (e.g., spouse, family members, mentors, friends)?

5. Given my age, how many more years do I need to continue to work? How many more years do I want to work regardless of income?

6. Do I have the support of my key loved ones? If not, how can I best go about getting that support?

7. What is my calling in life? Am I following it?

8. What is really important to me: what are my specific values and what is my purpose?

9. What am I passionate about? What are my marketable skills?

10. What aspects of work bring me joy and satisfaction, and what aspects of my work do I dislike and wish to give up?

11. What activities consistently yield personal meaning for me, in or out of the work place?

12. How will I continue to find personal meaning, a sense of personal contribution, and personal connection to others once I retire from the practice of medicine?

13. What legacy do I wish to leave in this world?

Success in Stages 3 and 4 requires that you clearly identify your personal values, personal purpose, sense of calling, and unique skills and abilities that have value in the marketplace—answering these questions can help you do that. By using and integrating this knowledge of yourself, you eventually are able to craft a new vision for your career or for retirement—one that is filled with passion, commitment, and is well integrated with your deeper values.

Of all the questions above, the ones pertaining to values, purpose, calling, and meaning are the most important and the most difficult for physicians to answer. They are questions that probe the soul and the spirit of the individual.

Answers require time alone to think and to reflect. Meaningful answers will come more easily and more quickly to those who seek help from mentors, certified career coaches familiar with the lives and challenges of physicians, therapists, and family and intimate friends. Those who are successful learn to be patient and wait for the answers to become manifest. Rushing this phase of transition usually leads to a poor career decision—one that is not consonant with your inner self.

Those choosing to cocoon will begin to do the self-exploring mentioned earlier and have lots of time to answer all of these questions. Those choosing the mini-transition will usually spend less time on the deeper questions, using the more practical questions to begin planning specific action steps to reengineer their work and/or obtain new skills/training.

3. Taking the Leap of Faith

The third stage of transition is the actual process of activating a plan for a mini-transition or a full-life transition created in Stage 2. In this third phase, specific steps propel you toward the future you envision for yourself. Action steps should be "SMART": Specific, Measurable, Achievable, Relevant, and Time-specific. My experience is that physicians in this stage benefit from having a career coach or mentor to help them formulate their action steps and help them stay on target and be accountable.

During both mini-transitions and full-life transitions, you can anticipate Stage 3 to be stressful. Therefore, first and foremost, ensure a sensible self-care plan is in place. Ideally that plan includes regular aerobic exercise at least 30 minutes three days a week, at least 50 hours of sleep a week, a healthy diet, a program of regular spirituality, and time for friends and fun. Such a plan for life balance is the most powerful form of stress busting available. (See Chapter 7.)

Now is the time to implement values-based time management and values-based money management strategies with professional support as needed. This may include a career/life coach and/or a certified financial planner.

Those who have been down this path successfully recommend that you engage in continuous learning, explore your fondest dreams and wishes without internal judgment or self-criticism, learn to ask for help, and finally, never look back! Above all else, transition is a spiritual path that requires a leap of faith, trust in yourself, and willingness to act despite your fear and inability to predict the outcome.

PITFALLS AND KEYS TO SUCCESS

In addition to courage, successful medical career transitions require patience, self-reflection, and the help of others. A good support network is critical, as well as skills in self-nurturing and self-care. Full-life transitions require, on average, three years, although this is highly variable and can be shortened with the assistance of an effective mentor or career coach. In my experience, the most common pitfall encountered by physicians in transition is expecting themselves to do it too quickly and then regretting a too-quick decision.

There is danger in seeking a "quick fix." Jumping quickly into an MPH or MBA program, or the hottest new consulting field, while tempting, may not be a suitable choice for you. Take the time to identify a new career path that reflects your personal values, interests, personality, motivated skills, and personal sense of purpose or calling. Remember, if you are having a problem making a career decision, you didn't get into the conundrum overnight. Neither can you expect to resolve it with the snap of a finger.

Avoiding activities that increase your self-awareness is a sure prescription for a failed transition. Rather, look within and plan your new career from the inside out. Once you are clear about your purpose, career values, unique skills, and passions, set about to align this inner work with new outer work.

Don't be in too big a hurry to leave clinical medicine. Many physicians I have coached initially wanted to leave clinical medicine, but subsequently found that addressing their issues with burnout and poor work-life balance successfully restored their enjoyment of clinical practice.

Finally, move forward despite your fear of the unknown, develop a willingness to let go of outcomes and you can expect thrilling times ahead.

References

1. Shanafelt,TA, Boone S, Litjen T, et. al. Burnout and satisfaction with work-life balance among US physicians relative to the general population. *Arch Int Med.* 2012;172(18):1377–1385.
2. Hudson, FM, and McLean, PD. Life launch: *A passionate guide to the test of your life.* Santa Barbara, CA: The Hudson Institute Press;, 1995.
3. Bridges, W. *Transitions. Making sense of life's changes.* Reading, MA: Addison-Wesley Publishing Co.; 1980.
4. Kubler-Ross, E. *On death and dying.* New York: The MacMillan Co.; 1969.

Resources

Block, D and Richmond, L. Soul work. *Finding the work you love, loving the work you have.* Palo Alto, CA: Davies Black Publishing; 1998.

Moskowitz, PS, Blau JM, Harris, SM, and Paprocki, RJ. *Medical practice divorce: Successfully managing a medical practice breakup.* Chicago: American Medical Association Press; 2001.

Moskowitz, PS. Physician renewal: The importance of life balance. *Career Planning and Adult Development Journal.* 14(1);81–92. Spring 1998.

Needleman, J. *Money and the meaning of life.* New York: Doubleday; 1991.

Notman, MT. Physician temperament, psychology, and stress. In: Goldman LS, Myers, M, Dickstein LJ. *The Handbook of Physician Health.* Chicago: American Medical Association Press; 2000; 39–51.

Snyder M and Zvenko, D. Physician burnout project. Project Report. Sacramento: Sacramento-El Dorado Medical Society; 1997.

The Mid-Career Physician

CHAPTER 9

Growing, Marketing, and Creating the Ideal Medical Practice

Neil H. Baum, MD

PHYSICIANS AT ALL STAGES IN their careers have an opportunity to develop their ideal medical practice. Beginning physicians may take advantage of marketing strategies to build their practices, but probably are better served by becoming comfortable in the practice, learning the technology, and if they are specialists, generating referrals from other physicians in the community. Retiring physicians are comfortable with the status quo and want to keep their practice going without much additional effort or may be looking for ways to decrease their patient load and patient responsibilities.

This chapter focuses on mid-career physicians and how they can use marketing techniques to create the ideal medical practice. There are four pillars to a successful medical practice:

1. Keeping and educating current patients;
2. Attracting new patients;
3. Enhancing communication with physicians; and
4. Motivating your staff.

No pillar is more important than the others; all four are necessary to guarantee success.

PILLAR 1: KEEPING AND EDUCATING CURRENT PATIENTS

It's nice to get new patients, but it's more important to keep the ones you already have. In most professions and businesses, the cost of keeping an established customer is one-fifth the cost of acquiring a new one. Medical practices are no exception. The patients you have right now are the backbone of your practice. If you are not doing a good job with the patients you already have, spending thousands of dollars on a marketing plan to bring in new patients is pointless.

> ### *Thank you for helping us to serve you better!*
>
> Was it easy for you to get an appointment in this office?
> ____ Yes   ____ No
>
> Is your general impression of this office favorable?
> ____ Yes   ____ No
>
> Was the office staff friendly and concerned?
> ____ Yes   ____ No
>
> Did the doctor adequately answer your questions?
> ____ Yes   ____ No
>
> Would you recommend this office to someone else?
> ____ Yes   ____ No
>
> Do you have any additional comments?

Figure 9-1. Patient Survey Card

Look at your practice from your patients' perspective. It is critical to know the needs and expectations of your patients and your referring physicians. The best way to do this is by asking your patients what they think about the various aspects of your practice; this also will reveal your practice's strengths and weaknesses. Even practices that are full should periodically evaluate their services and listen to their patients—the cup may not "runneth over" forever.

Tom Peters, the nationally renowned author of In Search of Excellence, describes two keys to success in business:

- Find out what the customer (patient) wants and give him or her more of it; and
- Find out what the customer (patient) does not want and be sure to avoid it.

Gather information about your patients' perspective. Here are five effective techniques for determining how patients perceive your practice and for evaluating your performance and reputation:

1. Conduct personal interviews.
2. Conduct patient surveys.
3. Create a focus group.
4. Use a suggestion box.
5. Commission evaluation by a mystery shopper.

Although I have used all five techniques, my favorite and the most cost-effective involves a survey card that is given to every patient on every office visit (Figure 9-1) when he or she checks in. The patient can complete the survey in the reception area or exam room and return it to the receptionist before leaving the practice.

Neil Baum, M.D.
UROLOGY

What three questions would you like answered today?

1. _____
   _____

2. _____
   _____

3. _____
   _____

Please complete the back of this card.

Figure 9-2. Questions to Ask the Doctor

A nurse or the medical assistant reviews the cards and responds to negative comments with a phone call. If necessary, I respond to the patient's complaint.

There is another benefit to the survey card. The reverse side of the card prompts patients to write down the three questions they would like you to address during their current visit to the office (Figure 9-2). This deters last-minute discussions, often after you have closed the chart or electronic medical record, that you don't have time to address adequately. Since my office has implemented use of this survey card, we seldom get follow-up phone calls from patients about issues they forgot to ask about. The survey card demonstrates that we care about the patients and want to be certain to answer all their questions at the time of their office visit.

Develop an on-time practice philosophy. According to the most common complaint patients have about the healthcare experience is "waiting for the doctor."[1] Spending time in the reception area probably accounts for more patient dissatisfaction than any other aspect of medical care. According to one survey,[2] nearly one in four patients claimed to have waited 30 minutes or longer before seeing the doctor.

To get an accurate picture of the schedule in your practice, conduct a "time and motion" study. For 3–5 days, place a sheet on each patient's record or superbill and log in the following:

- Time of the appointment;
- Time the patient arrived;
- Time the patient left the office; and

- How much time the patient spent with the physician.

You will be amazed to discover that patients are waiting 1–2 hours to see the physician, and the physician is spending only 5 minutes with the patient.

By conducting a time and motion study, you will discover that there are predictable periods when backlogs occur. Often, these delays are the result of "working a patient into" the schedule. Unscheduled patients who are told to come in without an appointment inevitably displace already scheduled patients and delay their visit.

One way to avoid this scenario is to create "sacred" time slots. These are 15-minute intervals at the end of the morning or afternoon in which unscheduled patients can be worked into the round of visits. Instead of telling the patient to "just come in," I tell them to report at a specific time. We do not fill these time slots with routine appointments and we do not fill them prior to 9:00 a.m. each day. This leaves two or three slots open for patients who must be seen that day.

Few physicians can change healthcare policy. But all of us can be more sensitive to our patients' time and make an effort to see them as soon as possible, thereby eliminating one of patients' most common complaints: the long wait to see their doctor.

Talk to the patient and not the computer. The number of physicians who have adopted electronic health records (EHRs) has doubled since 2008. Though the potential for this technology to improve healthcare is great, EHRs could be the source of a communication breakdown between patients and physicians.[3]

One of the most common complaints that doctors hear from their patients is that the doctor looks at the computer instead of the patient. We need to increase the time with the patient and decrease the time with the computer. We need to relate on a human level, not electronically.

A drawing created by a young pediatric patient that appeared in JAMA in 2012 shows a pediatric patient sitting on the table with her mother beside her. Her sister is on the right side of the drawing holding a baby. And where is the doctor? He is looking at his computer with his back to the patient and her family. This is not a way to build rapport or enhance communication. This is a problem for most physicians who have adopted electronic medical records (EMRs).

One solution is to make use of a scribe—a person who shadows a physician and records the findings on the computer, thus freeing the doctor to have more eye-to-eye contact with the patient. Another benefit of using a scribe is that the doctor does not have to touch the computer or the keyboard, which is very attractive to mid-career physicians who may not have grown up with touchpads and tablets.

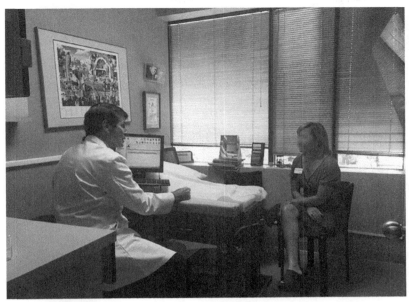

Figure 9-3. Effective Office Configuration

If you are not able to avail yourself of a scribe, at least look at the patient and the computer at the same time. Figure 9-3 is an example of my office configuration; it allows me to look at the computer and the patient at the same time.

Pick up the telephone and reach out. The most effective way to provide patients with a memorable experience is by taking a few minutes to call them at home. Which patients should you call? Call patients who are undergoing outpatient studies or procedures, those recently discharged from the hospital, and those who require a little more hand holding and attention. You can be sure that every patient who undergoes a procedure or is discharged from the hospital has questions about the findings, precautions, medications, and follow-up. A call from a nurse or doctor helps allay their apprehension and stress and often keeps them from calling the office with questions and concerns.

My nurse or medical assistant identifies key patients and contacts them at the end of the workday. She is usually able to answer all the questions but may identify two or three that require my attention. She tells the patient what time I will call so the patient can keep the phone line free.

Calling patients usually takes no more than 5 to 10 minutes a day and provides me with great satisfaction. Patients are usually shocked—and happy—that their physician is calling them at home. The advantages of this strategy include:

- Fewer calls from your patients;
- More efficient use of your time; and

- Deep appreciation by the patient.

One patient I called at home wrote me a note that I think is worth mentioning: "This is the first time a member of your profession has taken the time to call me at home and check on my condition. Undoubtedly, it will foster a better relationship between you and me."

PILLAR 2: ATTRACTING NEW PATIENTS

External marketing—getting the word out to the public—makes some doctors uncomfortable, it takes them out of their comfort zone. Some doctors think "marketing" is synonymous with "advertising."

The essence of external marketing is speaking and writing to increase your visibility among your peers and in the community. These techniques do not require large amounts of money, additional staff, or more than minimal assistance from your hospital public relations and marketing departments.

Present to the public. Few of us are naturally gifted public speakers, but if you acquire effective public speaking skills and begin giving presentations about your areas of expertise, you will be amazed at the increased demand for your presentations and the commensurate number of new patients filling your appointment book. When you take your message to the podium, audiences have an opportunity to not only learn more about your medical topic and how it applies to their health and wellness, but to interact with you.

If you want to do public speaking, you should generate interest in your speaking engagements. Contact the meeting planners at local churches, service organizations such as Lions Clubs and Rotary, and patient advocacy organizations such as the American Cancer Society, American Diabetes Association, and American Heart Association. You can get a list of these organizations and clubs from the local Chamber of Commerce.

I created a public relations packet that I sent to meeting planners in the community. The packet included a brief biography that outlined my credentials, a list of organizations or groups to whom I had given talks in the past, and a few testimonials from previous audience members. I also included a fact sheet (Figure 9-4) and several articles about the topic to be covered. The articles were written by me for local outlets or were written by others for publication in national magazines or other publications.

After your talk, be available to answer questions. Have plenty of business cards to hand out as well as your practice brochure and articles that pertain to the topic you presented.

Dr. Neil Baum
3525 Prytania, New Orleans, LA
FAQs on the Enlarged Prostate

What is BPH?
Benign prostatic hyperplasia is commonly known as enlarged prostate. BPH is a non-cancerous condition in which prostate cells grow, enlarging the gland and causing it to squeeze the urethra. A variety of symptoms may result, including difficult, frequent or urgent urination.

When should I seek BPH treatment?
If you are experiencing BPH symptoms that are affecting your quality of life, such as losing sleep because you need to wake during the night to urinate, you are unable to urinate, you are unable to delay urination, have hesitancy, or a weak urine stream, check with your urologist to discuss if it is time to seek treatment.

BPH is not cancerous and is not life threatening, but it does create bothersome symptoms can significantly impact quality of life.

What are the long-term risks of BPH?
If left untreated, BPH can progress and cause subsequent medical issues. When the bladder does not empty completely, you become at risk for developing urinary tract infections. Other serious problems can also develop over time, including bladder stones, blood in the urine (hematuria), incontinence, or urinary retention. In rare cases, bladder and/or kidney damage can develop from BPH.

What are the treatment options?
Based on the AUA Guidelines for the treatment of BPH, there are four recommended treatment options: Watchful waiting, medications, in-office therapy, and surgery.

Are in-office therapies safe?
Yes, these treatments are safe. UroLift has been cleared by the FDA to treat BPH. In-office BPH treatments are associated with few side effects and adverse events.

Are in-office therapies effective?
Based on clinical studies, in-office procedures is proven to be a safe, effective and durable option for BPH with very few side effects.

Are in-office therapies covered by insurance?
Medicare and many commercial insurance plans provide coverage for the UroLift procedure. Ask your doctor's office to assist you by providing the information your insurance plan may require.

Do in-office therapies hurt?
Some men describe the UroLift as causing some discomfort, while most men report no discomfort at all.

Will I need a catheter after the treatment?
Most patients will not need a catheter after the procedure.

Can I go home right after the procedure?
Yes. You should arrange for someone to drive you home because you may have been given some medication to help you relax during the procedure. Your urologist will give you post-treatment instructions and prescriptions and explain the recovery period to you.

Bottom Line: BPH is a common problem and effective treatments are available. For more answers, speak to your physician.

Figure 9-4. Example of a Fact Sheet

Facilitate support groups. Conducting a support group is an excellent way to target patients who have a specific diagnosis or disease state. It's easy to start a support group with patients in your practice. Organize a meeting and encourage them to invite others whom they think may be interested. Identify others who have a chronic problem—perhaps someone who attended your presentation—and invite them to a meeting of the support group. They will appreciate your interest and expertise and may become patients in your practice. Potential patients get to know who you are, what you do, and where to find you.

As you schedule your meeting, select a date two or three months in the future and identify several alternative dates. Tuesday or Wednesday evenings are the best nights for meetings, as most people will not have conflicting events in the middle of the week. However, if your target audience members are senior citizens, they may not be able to attend or drive at night; in that case, a Saturday morning or weekday afternoon meeting might be better.

I also recommend you provide a sign-in sheet to record the names and email addresses of all attendees. Within one week after the support group presentation, you can send a follow-up email and appropriate additional information to those on your sign-in sheet. The email should thank them for attending and let them know you are available to answer any questions. Add the attendees to your database and periodically contact them through newsletters and emails when new treatments or diagnostic techniques are available.

Market to immigrant and ethnic communities. You have an advantage in attracting non-English-speaking members of the community if you can speak their language. Identify the predominant language of your target patients and try to learn some basics of their language, such as greetings, farewells, and names of body parts. This not only will make diagnoses more efficient, it will also make your patients feel welcomed. You also can serve their needs if someone on your staff can translate.

Provide translations of your educational materials for your patients who are more comfortable with a language besides English. If these are not already available from pharmaceutical or medical manufacturing companies, have the most frequently used materials translated into their language. Professional medical interpreters advise it is best to employ a trained medical professional with medical experience to translate the materials. Without specific training in the language and the nuances of translating during a medical examination, diagnostic cues and treatment recommendations can be missed or misinterpreted. Figure 9-5 provides a list of translation services that specialize in medicine.

Be sure to include information on your website and other social media that you accept patients who speak other languages.

> **American Translators Association (ATA):** www.atanet.org
>
> **Society of Medical Interpreters (SOMI):** www.sominet.org
>
> **National Council on Interpreting in Health Care (NHIC):** www.ncihc.org
>
> **The National Board of Certification for Medical Interpreters:** http://www.certifiedmedicalinterpreters.org/resources
>
> **International Medical Interpreters Association (IMIA):** www.imiaweb.org

Figure 9-5. Medical Translation Resources

Write articles for consumer publications. How many referrals or new patients do you receive from the articles you have written for professional journals? There is a good chance your answer is the same as mine: "none." My CV lists more than 200 articles I have published in peer-reviewed professional journals, yet I have not seen a single referral or a new patient as a result of these articles.

However, I have written several thousand articles for local newspapers and magazines that have generated hundreds of new patient visits to my practice. By writing articles for local newspapers and magazines, you can effectively promote your practice and your areas of interest and expertise. Published bylined articles in the lay press increase your visibility, credibility, and, ultimately, profitability. People are more likely to believe you if you have been published.

By writing articles for the local press, you can become a media resource. Reporters and editors will contact you for articles or ask you for quotations to include in articles they are writing. And, if you are responsive, they will keep you in their databases as a content person to call on whenever your specialty is in the news.

You can do your part to promote this visibility as well. For example, when Whoopi Goldberg shared her experience with urinary incontinence on "The View," I contacted the local paper and offered to provide information about the problem of incontinence and overactive bladder and how an outpatient evaluation can often result in cure of this disease.

In addition to addressing popular topics such as nutrition and cancer prevention, you can create an interesting article about new procedures, new treatments, a unique case with an excellent result, or the use of new technologies.

Like medical skills, speaking and writing skills can be learned and polished. The more you do, the better you get. The better you get, the more patients you will attract to your practice.

PILLAR 3: COMMUNICATING WITH REFERRING PHYSICIANS

Presentations about marketing a medical practice often focus on the three As: availability, affability, and affordability. Since all physicians think of themselves as available, as likeable, and as offering appropriately priced services, how do you differentiate yourself from the competition? Just using fancy stationary, a slick three-color brochure, a practice logo, or a website will not do the trick. Let the truth be told: the last things you need are a brochure, fancy stationery, and a logo.

One of the biggest misconceptions about marketing is that to do it well, you must spend lots of money on peripherals. There are many far more effective and essential steps to marketing than running radio, TV, and print media campaigns.

The most essential element of your marketing plan is a practice that is user-friendly and patient-centric. Nowhere is this more important than in the area of working with your colleagues who are capable and currently referring patients. Here are nine techniques that will enhance your relationships with your fellow physicians.

1. Write an effective referral letter. According to the *Annals of Family Medicine*[4] more than 50% of physicians state that effective communication is the reason they refer their patients to a specific doctor. Here are the other reasons physicians refer patients to colleagues:

- Return pt. to PCP: 100%
- Medical skill: 88%
- Access to the practice and acceptance of insurance: 55%
- Previous experience with the specialist: 59%
- Quality of communication: 53%
- Board certification of specialist: 33%
- Medical school, residency: <10%

When you have been referred a patient, your goal should be for the referring physician to receive your referral letter—the follow-up report—before the patient calls or sees the referring physician again.

Effective referral letters are short. The referring doctor is not interested in the nuances of your history or the fine details of your physical exam. The key ingredients are: 1) diagnosis, 2) medications you have prescribed for the patient, and 3) your treatment plan.

For example, Dr. Bill Smith refers Jane Doe who has an overactive bladder and a cystocele. Her urinalysis is negative, so you prescribe an anticholinergic agent and plan to see the patient in one month to do a symptom check and possibly

Dear Bill,

Jane Doe was seen for a problem of overactive bladder. I recommended <name of medication>, 5mg/day. I plan to obtain a urodynamic study and cystoscopy if she does not improve on smooth muscle relaxants.

I will keep in touch with you regarding her urologic progress.

Sincerely,

Neil Baum

Figure 9-6. Referral Letter to Referring Physician

a urodynamic study if she is not better. The letter can be faxed to the referring doctor before the patient leaves the office and you can be certain that it will arrive before the patient calls the doctor with questions or concerns. Figure 9-6 illustrates a possible referral letter.

EMRs can fax the entire note to the referring physician, although physicians typically don't want to see the entire letter. Most EMRs will allow you to select fields that contain the diagnosis, the medications prescribed, and the treatment plan.

By keeping referring physicians informed, you help them captain the patient's healthcare ship.

2. Personally meet every physician who refers a patient. That means meeting all of them, not just your long-standing referral sources. Make an effort to reach out to new physicians and tell them about your areas of interest or expertise.

3. Refer new patients to referring physicians. If you are a mid-career physician, don't use the same colleagues repeatedly. If a doctor is sending you new patients, it is in your best interest to reverse-refer when a patient needs the services of that specialist. You can be sure these referring doctors will appreciate your referrals.

4. Recognize and acknowledge accomplishments of referring physicians and of their family members. If one of your referring physicians has received an honor or an award, send him or her a congratulatory note. Also, if a referring physician's children have accomplished an academic or athletic achievement, acknowledge this achievement with a note. They will appreciate your taking the time to send a personal note.

5. Share information with a no-meeting journal club. It is challenging to keep up with the literature in your own specialty, let alone articles appearing in other medical publications. One of the easiest ways to stay current on the literature is to copy articles that may be of interest to your colleagues and target their reading by placing a sticky note where you would like them to look so they don't have to read the entire article.

6. Share non-medical as well as medical information. Share non-medical information with your colleagues and let them know you are thinking of them even when you are not discussing patient care. For example, one of my colleagues collects fine pens. I saw an article about a very expensive pen made with diamonds and sent the story to my friend, suggesting that he might tell his wife what was on his wish list.

7. Keep the referring doctor in the medical loop. If you are caring for a patient and plan to discharge the patient, make sure you or someone in your office contacts the referring doctor and informs him or her that the patient is being discharged so he or she doesn't make unnecessary rounds on the patient. Also notify referring doctors when you admit their patients to the hospital, after surgery or a procedure, or when you have a significant lab/path report.

8. Thank ER doctors for referring patients to your practice. Even if you are a mid-career physician and are not seeking referrals from the ER, it is such a nice gesture to send a note to ER doctors after seeing a referred patient to let them know what you found on the follow-up exam and compliment the doctor on the management of the patient. This may be the only referral note an ER doctor ever receives.

9. Don't forget non-physician referral sources. Non-physician referrals include nurses, pharmacists, pharmaceutical representatives, social workers, lawyers, beauticians, and manicurists. Many of these non-physicians can send patients to physicians.

No matter how successful a mid-career physician is, he or she needs to be cognizant of the importance of communicating with colleagues. The communication can help establish a collegial relationship with fellow colleagues that can enhance our practices.

PILLAR 4: MOTIVATING STAFF

The success of any medical practice begins and ends with the staff. You can have new patients, excellent relationships with your referring physicians, and a plentiful number of existing patients, but if you don't have a staff that is excited, enthusiastic, and knowledgeable when answering the telephone and dealing with patients, your ability to grow your practice will be ineffective.

Create a Mission Statement. Nearly every successful business and every successful medical practice has a well-defined vision, mission, goal, or objective. The mission statement should spell out the purpose of the practice and the methods of achieving that purpose. It serves as the road map that provides direction to all of the members of the staff—doctors included.

This is our mission statement:

We are committed to:

Excellence,

Providing the best urologic healthcare for our patients, and

The persistent and consistent attention to the LITTLE details because they make a BIG difference.

The mission statement is posted in prominent places in the office (in the reception area and in most of the examination rooms) to remind the staff and our patients of our dedication to excellent customer service. It is also featured prominently on the website and on a large banner in the employee lounge.

Develop a Policy Manual. Every practice needs a manual that includes its rules and regulations. The manual should cover job descriptions, dress codes, hours of operation, division of office responsibilities, vacation days, sick days, and emergency telephone numbers. Ideally, this manual should serve as a guide for any new or temporary employees who come to work in the office.

We summarize our policy manual with this expectation:

Rule 1: The patient is always right.

Rule 2: If you think the patient is wrong, reread Rule 1.

All other policies are null and void.

Whenever a mistake or problem occurs, the first question we ask each other is, "Did we adhere to the mission statement and the policy statement?" Usually we discover that we did not. We use the mission statement and the policy manual statement to refocus on our number one priority: our patients.

No-Cost Techniques to Motivate Staff

A motivated staff will create an effective team environment. Most enlightened businesses see that team management leads to increased output and productivity. Your employees want to be valued as human beings and individuals, not just as workers. The more you include employees in the process of running the office, the more invested they become in helping to improve it.

What do you like the most about this job?

What would you like to improve?

Where do you want to be professionally in the next 3, 6, 12 months?

What can I do to help you reach your goals?

Figure 9-7. Employee Performance Review Worksheet

Have a Performance Review. Employees like to know where they stand and how they can improve performance on the job. Staff members want feedback on their progress or even lack of progress. The best way to furnish this important feedback is with periodic performance reviews. I suggest meeting with your employees on a scheduled basis—about every 3–4 months.

Each employee is given a worksheet to complete before the scheduled review (Figure 9-7). I end each performance review on a positive note. I tell the employees how valued they are and how much of an asset they are to the practice. Of course, these meetings should be documented in the employees' files.

Encourage Continuing Education. Like you, your staff members require continuing motivational experiences. It is a favorable return on your investment to encourage your staff to participate in continuing education courses and it is necessary to support their efforts financially. Offer to pay the fees when your employees take seminars and classes. Suggest that your employees take courses in computers, social media, marketing, or anything else that will help the practice grow and prosper.

Empower Your Staff. Office management is complicated. Few doctors have a thorough understanding of all of the business aspects of a medical practice. Most successful physicians have learned to empower their employees to take control and assume responsibility for their decisions and actions.

In my office, I empower any employee to make financial decisions up to $200 without consulting with the doctors. If the office needs a new telephone answering machine, I want my employees to consider which features we need, check the ones that are available, and compare prices at the local electronic outlet, office supply stores, and on Amazon.com to find the best machine at the lowest price.

Promote a Positive Mental Attitude. As Ralph Waldo Emerson once said, "Nothing great was ever achieved without enthusiasm." This is also true in the practice of medicine. When the doctor has a positive mental attitude, the employees are motivated by example. If, on the other hand, the doctor is easily irritated,

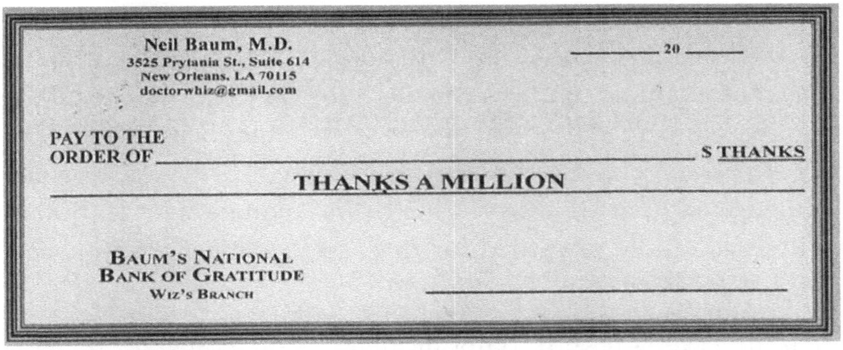

Figure 9-8. Thanks a Million Check

brings personal problems to work, and takes it out on the employees, they, in turn, will take it out on the patients.

Employees are on stage from the moment they walk in the door in the morning, so they must leave all other problems and concerns on the other side of the door. They must recognize that they are responsible for ensuring that each patient has a positive experience with the office at every contact point with the practice. That includes the telephone system, the receptionist who welcomes the patient to the practice, the nurse taking the patient into the exam room, the billing clerk who discusses the patient's bill, and, yes, the doctor, too! We all contribute to the patient's experience and we all must have a positive attitude.

Recognize Achievement. Nothing is more motivating for employees than for the doctor to recognize their accomplishments. When you see improvement in job performance, tell the person directly—you will be improving that employee's self-esteem. This improves the employee's confidence and also helps him or her improve the self-esteem of fellow employees.

Show Your Staff That You Care. Your employees need to know that you care about them not just as workers, but as individuals. When any of my employees or their family members are sick, I call them at home to check on them and make sure they have access to adequate medical care. If someone gets sick in the office, I call another medical office and get the employee seen immediately.

Catch Your Staff Doing Things Right. My philosophy is to praise in public, pan in private. When I catch an employee doing something right, I send a thank-you note to the employee's home address, making sure that it arrives on a Saturday. Hopefully, the employee will show my note to family and friends. I use a specially created card or "Thanks a Million Check" (Figure 9-8). You will be amazed at how appreciative employees are that you not only recognized their superior service, but that you also took the time to put it writing.

Reward Your Staff for Saving Money or Reducing Overhead Expenses. If one of your staff members comes up with an idea that saves the practice money, give a bonus. For example, the 15-year-old autoclave broke down. When I tried to get parts, I was informed that machine was no longer being made. The nurse in our office took the autoclave to the hospital's biomedical engineering department, which installed a $30 part that saved me from buying a new $2,000 autoclave. The nurse deserved to be rewarded for that, so I gave her a $50 check right on the spot.

I am trying to motivate my staff to not just earn more money for the practice, but to reduce expenses as well. They are paid for identifying and designing money-saving ideas.

Include Your Staff in the Decision-Making Process. Ask your employees for advice, then make sure you use it. Your staff members are on the front line and they want the office routine to go well. You must include them in the decision-making process, whether the task is writing a mission statement or policy manual, determining a change in procedures, implementing an EMR, or meeting new job candidates. By including them, you are making them feel part of the team.

Have Fun with Your Staff. Whenever you can provide an unexpected perk for your staff, they will appreciate the gesture. For example, one week we had two employees who were unable to work: one was on vacation and the other was ill at home. We had to work harder to take up the slack for five days. In spite of being shorthanded, we were able to function at regular speed and capacity without affecting the quality of care that we provided our patients. I was so impressed with the extra effort that I arranged for a massage therapist to visit our practice at the end of the day on Friday and give everyone a 20-minute massage as a way of saying thank you.

The fourth pillar encourages your staff to develop a team spirit and this makes good business sense. When your employees have a personal investment in creating a positive experience for the patients, they will go the extra mile for your patients and for your practice.

THE FINAL BOTTOM LINE

Mid-career physicians can certainly build a practice by word of mouth and doing a great job caring for the patients in their practices, hoping patients will tell others about their positive experience with the practice. Try a few of these ideas and you will find that you can have the exact kind of practice that you enjoy and are proud to be a member of. It will put you on the road to developing the ideal medical practice.

Word of mouth was the time-honored method of attracting new patients for thousands of years. That method still works today. Ensuring that your patients have an outstanding experience during their visit is one of the smartest strategies to market and promote your practice. Just like a table with four legs is stable, your practice has the greatest potential for success when it is supported by the four pillars described in this chapter.

References

1. Press Ganey Associates. 2011. 2011 Pulse Report: Perspectives on American Health Care. South Bend, IN.: Press Ganey.
2. Rappleye E. March 26, 2015. How long is the average wait at a physician's office? *Beckers Hospital Review.*
3. Dolan PL. July 23, 2012. How to communicate well with a patient while working on an EHR. American Medical Association. amednews.com. *http://www.amednews.com/article/20120723/ business/307239968/5/)*
4. Kinchen KS, Cooper LA, Levine D, Wang NY, Powe NR. Referral of patients to specialists: factors affecting choice of specialist by primary care physicians. *Ann Fam Med.* 2004 May-Jun;2(3):245–52.

CHAPTER 10

Risk Management, Estate Planning, and Investing

Joel M. Blau and Ronald J. Paprocki

RISK MANAGEMENT, IN THE CONTEXT of a properly structured financial plan, focuses on the task of controlling that which cannot be controlled. Other than liability issues, it is important to protect against the two major hazards: death and disability. Much time and money are invested in many different areas of insurance, from malpractice insurance to health insurance to auto insurance and homeowners insurance. Unfortunately, very little time is spent protecting a physician's most important asset: the ability to earn income. Much of this lack of attention is due in part to the way life and disability insurance are purchased.

The insurance agent's job is to sell you the greatest amount of insurance you will buy, with very little attention to your specific goals and objectives. So, it is imperative physicians have a general understanding of how these unique insurance products can be used to meet the risk-protection needs of an overall financial plan. Refer to Chapter 6 for "Insuring Your Future."

ESTATE PLANNING

Estate tax planning is an important element of the financial planning process. Why work so hard to accumulate assets and then let the government take up to 40% in estate taxes? Why leave assets that were well-managed throughout your life in a state of confusion when you pass away?

The key objective of an estate plan is to maximize the available strategies in order to best preserve and manage your estate. Understand that estate tax planning is truly a selfless endeavor because you may not receive a monetary benefit, but others certainly can. Also keep in mind that for married couples, the estate tax is typically deferred until the second death. Estate tax planning is not just about strategies that will leave more of the estate to your spouse, although as you will see, this can easily be accomplished.

You must take the time necessary to develop an efficient and psychologically comfortable estate plan. Take the time to consider the multitude of options available so you won't be forced to make quick, uninformed decisions.

Goals

When you plan your estate, you may have numerous goals, including:

- The effective distribution of your assets, making certain that your property is transferred to the individuals you wish at the time you believe is appropriate.
- Providing needed income to surviving family members or other dependents.
- Arranging for the management of assets for surviving family members.
- Avoiding the administrative headache of probate and the resulting fees.

However, for many physicians, the primary common goal of estate planning is to minimize federal estate taxes. This is accomplished through the use of estate tax credits and available deductions. An efficient estate plan will utilize credits and deductions, but there is much more that can be done. You can have the finest trust documents drafted by a leading estate attorney, but if this is not coordinated with the titling of your assets, your expensive documents may prove worthless in terms of the purpose for which they were intended.

Despite all the reasons to create an effective estate plan, many physicians have not bothered to make any inroads in this important area for several reasons. For example, they may believe they do not have enough money to worry about. However, their estate tax is based on all assets they own or control, and when you add the value of all assets plus the death benefits of life insurance policies, it is fairly easy to reach rather substantial numbers quickly.

Or they may think they don't need to plan their estate because all assets are to be given to their spouse. Current tax laws make transfers between spouses quite tax-advantaged; however, while transferring all assets to a spouse may provide temporary tax relief, it usually increases the total tax liability over the long run. In addition, such a strategy often places the responsibility of distribution of assets and the timing of such distributions entirely on the surviving spouse's shoulders.

Some physicians claim they simply do not care what happens to their assets after their death. But would they be concerned if the government's share of their estate was the largest single distribution made when compared to the assets distributed to family? Are they willing to give up as much as 40% of their assets to the government in the form of estate taxes, not to mention income taxes from retirement plans?

Most commonly, physicians tell us they are just too busy to address these matters. We suggest they ask themselves if the two hours spent getting their estate plan squared away is worth the possible $1 million in taxes they can save their estate. That seems to be a reasonable pay back of time.

Estate-planning attorneys tell us that physicians often initiate estate plans from their death beds or, interestingly enough, right before they travel abroad—even though they had the trip planned months in advance. This doesn't give the physician or the attorney enough time to do the job right. The result is usually a quick and supposedly temporary document that will be updated as soon as the physician returns. It is simply a short-term solution for a long-term problem.

The Estate-Planning Process

As you begin the estate-planning process, the first step is to identify your beneficiaries—the people or organizations you care about. Very simply, who do you want to inherit your estate? If you are married, a logical choice (and in many states a legal requirement) is to include the spouse in this category. Identify the primary beneficiary, who is the person first in line to inherit, and then look beyond the primary beneficiary to the contingent beneficiary, who is the individual who will receive your property in the event your primary beneficiary predeceases you. Children, other relatives, friends, or charitable entities are often the contingent beneficiaries.

You will also need to give some thought to how your beneficiaries or contingent beneficiaries will receive assets upon your death—an important decision that is oftentimes overlooked. For a spouse, a lump sum may be appropriate. For those other than a spouse, you might consider providing for income for a certain period, with distributions of principal at certain ages or after a certain number of years after your death. This "staggered" distribution arrangement allows a beneficiary the opportunity to acquire a greater degree of financial maturity before the entire estate is distributed.

Next, inventory your assets. This inventory should include all your investment assets, retirement plans, the value of your home and other real estate, as well as personal property, including jewelry, collectibles, furnishings, vehicles, and boats. Also include the value of your practice as well as the death benefit of the life insurance policies you own.

Wills

Many physicians are surprised to learn that a will may be the least-important element in their estate plan. A valid will provides directions to your survivors as to how you would like to have your assets distributed at your death. Think of your will simply as a note you are writing to a judge requesting that certain things be completed. The drawback to using a will as your only estate-planning tool is that the will only controls the distribution of solely titled assets (or beneficiary-designated assets that are paid to the estate). In addition, all assets that are distributed through a will must be probated.

Most wills are written so that all assets are transferred to the surviving spouse (or to the children if there is no surviving spouse). This is often referred to as an "I love you" will, since all assets are made available to the survivor. However, the will makes assets available in a manner that maximizes the ultimate estate tax liability on the assets. For most physicians, a simple will is insufficient on its own, but when combined with other estate tax strategies, can make a lot of sense in ensuring an efficient estate tax plan.

Trusts

Despite their apparent complexity, trusts can be very useful in many aspects of estate planning. To understand trusts, you need to know who the players are and what they do.

- *Grantor.* This is the individual who transferred funds into the trust.
- *Trustee.* The trustee is supposed to ensure that the terms of the trust, as outlined by the grantor, are carried out.
- *Beneficiary.* The beneficiary is the person (or individuals) for whom the trust has been created. Often a minor, the beneficiary can also be a surviving spouse, adult child, or any individual who is in need of financial assistance (or supervision) after the death of the grantor.

Now let's examine a couple of different type of trusts often used for estate-planning purposes.

The first is a *testamentary* trust. This trust is usually part of a will and is created after the death of the grantor. With a testamentary trust, assets are passed through probate before being managed by the trust. The trust can then help divide assets for each beneficiary, manage assets, or distribute assets as required by the directions of the trust.

A *living trust*, also known as an *inter vivos* trust, is created during the life of the grantor. Assets are transferred into the trust and thus avoid probate at the time of death. As an added benefit, living trusts provide benefits during life, particularly in the event of the incompetency of the grantor.

A living trust identifies contingent trustees who are able to assume the role of trustee in the event the original trustee (usually the grantor) is unable to perform his or her duties. Such forethought will avoid the excessive legal costs required if a grantor is declared incompetent, since in such cases annual accountings to the court are required.

A trust can be an excellent way to control the management and distribution of assets. However, a trust only works to the extent that assets have been transferred into the trust. We've seen physicians who have spent hours in their attorney's office creating what they hoped would be the trust arrangement for their estate, only to put off transferring their assets into the trust—so the trust never really controls anything! If you bother to create a trust for your estate plan, make certain your assets are titled in the way necessary for the trust to work!

Effective Planning

The most effective estate plan uses a variety of strategies. By combining the proper documents and strategies, you are in the best position to accomplish all of your estate-planning objectives for the appropriate distribution, efficient administration, and necessary management of your estate assets.

In addition, you can be certain that you have done as much as possible to position your assets at the time of your death for maximum income generation for surviving family as well as the preservation of your estate assets from the impact of estate taxation.

RISK REDUCTION OF INVESTMENT PORTFOLIOS

Asset allocation creates a balance for your portfolio by investing in a variety of asset classes, such as stocks, bonds, and money markets. Each component is designed to provide certain characteristics for your portfolio.

Stocks offer the potential to earn attractive returns, but they entail more risk than some other types of investments. Bonds are an integral part of asset allocation because they generally provide more stability than equities. By including both bonds and equities in your portfolio, you seek to balance it. Cash assets, such as money markets, offer liquidity and a convenient "parking place" for cash intended for future investment opportunities.

Within these general classes are subcategories. For example, the equity class of assets can be further divided into U.S. large company stocks, U.S. small company stocks, and the stocks of international companies. Fixed income can be subcategorized by length of maturity and includes both U.S. and international bonds. Over time, these asset classes perform differently. This also applies to international stocks and bonds. Therefore, diversification among asset classes is important to maintain a consistent level of performance over time.

Another concept that is important to the efficient management of an investment portfolio is modern portfolio theory. Three basic premises of modern portfolio theory are worth considering in detail.

1. Markets are efficient. Over time, it is difficult for an individual investor to consistently "beat the market." Technology has created an environment that makes information instantly available to a potentially limitless number of investors.

2. Attention should be focused on the investment portfolio as a whole rather than on individual investments that make up the portfolio. Studies have shown that over 90% of the impact of an investment portfolio is a result of the selection of asset classes rather than the selection of a particular security or market timing.[1] Therefore, much of the energy spent trying to pick or time the purchase of the "best" stock, bond, or mutual fund is wasted. Individual investors would be better served by deciding on and monitoring a specific asset class selection among domestic and international asset classes.

3. At any given level of risk, there is a particular combination of asset classes that will maximize return. Therefore, not only is the selection of the type of asset class important, but determining the amount to be invested in each class will help to maximize return at a given level of risk.

REDUCING RISK

There are two ways to reduce the impact of risk: diversification and time. Your investment time frame may be long-term (retirement), medium-term (college funding), or short-term (purchasing a new home). The more time you devote to any given investment strategy, the more predictable your return on investments will be.

If the investment time period is fewer than three to five years, the appropriate strategy would be to invest primarily in fixed income (bonds) and cash equivalents (money markets or treasury bills). If, however, the time period is expected to exceed three to five, investing a portion of assets in equities would be reasonable. Periods of longer than five years have provided a much lower level of volatility for equities (stocks).

Once you have defined your investment goals and determined a time frame, your investment strategy can be accomplished by creating a diversified portfolio. You diversify your portfolio by combining various asset classes, blending high-return/high-risk asset classes with lower-return/lower-risk asset classes.

By concentrating on asset class selection, you can structure a portfolio and be relatively confident of its overall risk as well as its projected long-term return. A number of computer software programs can help with asset allocation number crunching. Many financial advisors can also assist you properly structure a portfolio based on your specific risk/return parameters.

Now think about your own investment plan. Are you spending the majority of time on issues that add very little to the bottom line, such as market timing or specific stock selection? Most investors do! Physicians buy into the "hot" tip, because it is being promoted as a money-making sure thing. They do this without a thought to its place in their portfolio. If you need to buy this hot stock or take advantage of a tip, do it with a limited amount of funds you have set aside for such risk taking. But do it only after having set up a truly diversified, well-funded portfolio, not at the expense of a diversified investment plan.

Unfortunately, this is not how most physicians structure their portfolios. Highly respected economists vary with regard to their market forecasts, as do the top stock analysts working at the country's largest brokerage firms. What is known for certain is that no one can predict consistently when market declines or rallies will occur. (It's easy to do so in hindsight, however.)

Once you have focused on the most important determinant of a portfolio's performance—asset class selection—you can structure a portfolio that will meet your specific needs. After deciding how your portfolio should be allocated among the various asset classes, you can begin funding your investment plan.

For funding purposes, dollar cost averaging (DCA) is a technique used to reduce risk. By using a DCA strategy, investors purchase securities on a regular, systematic basis. By investing a set amount each month, the average purchase price tends to offset market fluctuations. DCA does NOT, however, assure a profit or protect against market losses

With constant market volatility, an investor doesn't know whether shares are overpriced or underpriced at any given time. Using DCA, the investor purchases shares of a fund over an extended period of time, averaging out the high and low purchases. The investor buys some shares when prices are low and other shares when prices are high. Using this strategy, losses during market declines are limited while the ability to participate in bull market movements is maintained.

While this principle applies to any fluctuating security, it ideally is suited for mutual fund investing. Mutual funds provide diversification, professional management, and controlled expenses. As a general rule, mutual funds allow additional investments to be made as often as you like. Many funds allow automatic investments to be set up from your checking account or money market fund on a monthly basis.

So often, investors let their emotions and stock market information overload guide their buying and selling decisions and end up buying high and selling low. The automatic investment plan guarantees that feelings about the stock market are put on the sidelines as dollars buy additional shares at varying prices.

If the stock market would move in just one direction—up—then it would be better to invest in one lump sum. Unfortunately, the market moves in cycles and fluctuates daily. DCA will not guarantee you a profit, but it is appropriate for long-term saving purposes such as retirement and college education funding for your children. Risk may be reduced because purchases of mutual fund shares are certain to be made at a variety of share prices. Obviously this is not a get-rich-quick market timing strategy. It is simply an effective method for accumulating an investment portfolio at a reasonable cost.

SUMMARY

Managing risk is an integral aspect of achieving long-term financial independence. It starts with the uncontrollables, such as death, disability, and estate planning, and then works its way through the investment process. The key going forward is the recognition of the particular risks and the actions you can take now to reduce or eliminate those risks. By addressing the risks proactively, you will be in the best position to achieve overall financial success.

Reference

1. Ibbotson RG and Kapplan PD. 2000. Does asset allocation policy explain 40, 90, or 100 percent of performance? *Financial Analysts Journal.* 2000;56(1):26–33

CHAPTER 11

Understanding Retirement Plans

Joel M. Blau and Ronald J. Paprocki

SETTING THE COURSE for true financial independence requires proactive planning and focuses on areas physicians are able to control, as opposed to potentially unpredictable retirement income sources such as Social Security or a potential future inheritance. The key is to plan and take action now in order to avoid surprises down the road.

As more physicians become aware of their own need to plan for future retirement, income security and qualified retirement plans remain the logical starting point. A qualified retirement plan (QRP) is a congressionally approved tax shelter that has many major tax advantages. From the employer's standpoint, plan contributions are a tax deduction for income tax purposes. For the employee, earnings on the plan's investments accumulate on a tax-deferred basis, and since participants are often in a lower tax bracket at retirement, they may pay less tax on the distributions.

QRPs are generally classified as "defined benefit" or "defined contribution." Some plans may combine features of both types.

DEFINED BENEFIT PLANS

Defined benefit plans tend to favor older, highly compensated employees such as physicians who are close to retirement. That is because the employer (the physician) has fewer years over which to accumulate enough money to provide the promised benefit. Actuarial calculations are made to determine how much money must be contributed each year to accumulate the amount that is necessary in the future to keep the doctor in a lifestyle similar to his or her lifestyle prior to retirement. Interest rates, investment rates of return, and the age of participants will affect the calculation. The investment risk rests solely on the employer, who is required to fund the plan adequately each year, although the annual contribution can vary based on the plan's investment results. The future benefit received may be based on a flat percentage of compensation, a percentage that increases with the length of service, a percentage that changes at certain compensation levels, or a number of other variables.

A defined benefit plan offers many advantages to the employee. First, the plan is funded completely by the employer, and neither the contributions nor earnings are taxed to the employee while in the plan. Also, the employee has peace of mind knowing he or she will receive a future benefit. Many plans even allow an employee to borrow from the plan within certain strict guidelines.

The primary disadvantage of a defined benefit plan relates to younger participants. Younger employees generally receive a smaller portion of the total contribution, primarily because of the longer time period until their retirement.

From an employer's standpoint, some advantages of a defined benefit plan are:

- Long-term employees can be rewarded with a substantial retirement benefit even though they are close to retirement age;
- Forfeitures from terminating employees reduce future funding requirements for current employees; and
- Plan investments are directed solely by the employer.

Although it was once the qualified retirement plan of choice for many medical practices, the defined benefit plan has become much less popular because of the following disadvantages to the employer:

- In low-profit years, the employer is still obligated to make plan contributions;
- Investment risk rests solely with the employer; and
- Administration costs are higher than for defined contribution plans because an actuary must be retained to certify the reasonableness of the contribution and deduction.

Recent legislation has lifted other defined benefit plan obstacles, and its popularity is again on the rise. Defined benefit plans afford significant opportunities for contribution and deduction.

DEFINED CONTRIBUTION PLANS

Several variations of defined contribution plans are commonly used by medical practices: money purchase pension plans, profit-sharing plans, age-weighted profit-sharing plans, new comparability plans, 401(k) savings plans, and "simple" plans.

Money Purchase Pension Plans

In a money purchase pension plan, the employer contributes a specified percentage of the total participating employees' salaries each year. This contribution is allocated among the participants. Up to 25% of the participants' payroll can be contributed and deducted by the employer. Plan contributions can be based on total compensation, including bonuses and overtime pay. Maximum recognized compensation for 2016 is $265,000, which is indexed for inflation in future years. A participant's annual account contribution may not exceed the lesser of 100% of compensation or $53,000 per year, excluding "catch-up" contributions of $6,000 for those 50 years of age and older, for a total of $59,000.

Money purchase pension plans typically favor younger participants because they have a longer time period over which their accounts will grow. In many instances, they will share in plan forfeitures, which occur when participants leave the practice before they have become 100% vested. The non-vested forfeitures can be reallocated to the remaining participants, thus benefiting employees who remain in the plan the longest.

In addition to the deductibility of the contributions, there are other advantages for the employer:

- Contributions, as well as administrative costs, are known in advance;
- Contributions will rise as compensation rises, but they are controllable by both formula and absolute dollar amounts; and
- The employer can direct the investment portfolio, or the employees can self-direct their own portions of the plan.

The primary disadvantage to the employer concerns mandatory contributions; the employer is obligated to make contributions, even in years when the practice loses money. The primary disadvantage to the employee is the lack of a guarantee regarding the amount of retirement benefit, since the investment risk rests on the employee participant regardless of who directs the investments.

Money purchase pension plans have all but become extinct. Profit-sharing plans (see below) now allow for up to the same 25% of salary contributions, but on a year-by-year discretionary basis.

Profit-Sharing Plans

For greater employer flexibility, a profit-sharing plan may be the defined contribution plan of choice. Employer contributions to the plan need not be made every year. The maximum annual deduction is limited to 25% of compensation, with an individual recognized maximum compensation of $265,000 (as of January 1, 2016). Although annual contributions are generally discretionary, if there are profits, the employer is expected to make "substantial and recurring" contributions. As a rule of thumb, contributions in 3 out of 5 years or 5 out of 10 years will usually satisfy the IRS.

For employees, profit-sharing plans tend to favor younger participants. However, the down sides of a profit-sharing plan are similar to a money purchase pension plan. There are no guarantees as to the amount of future retirement benefits, and the investment risk rests on the employee. In addition, there is no assurance of the frequency and amount of employer contributions.

Advantages of a profit-sharing plan to the employer include:

- The plan gives an incentive to employees to be productive to maximize the profit potential of the practice;
- Contributions are completely flexible; and
- Forfeitures of terminating employees are reallocated among active participants, generally with a greater percentage allocated to the highest salaried participants, such as the physicians.

While contribution limits of profit-sharing plans are set at 25% of covered payroll, this type of plan will generally not produce as large a contribution and deduction for older employees when compared to a defined benefit plan.

Age-Weighted Profit-Sharing Plans

Since defined contribution plans tend to favor younger employees, another alternative is the age-weighted profit-sharing plan. Employer contributions in this type of plan are not necessarily based on profits; the contributions are totally flexible and at the discretion of the employer. Contributions need not be made yearly, as long as they are "substantial and recurring." Employer contributions are allocated to provide an equal retirement benefit at normal retirement age for all participants. Older participants are favored from a contribution perspective, since they are closer to retirement. However, all participants would receive the same projected retirement benefit percentage at age 65.

Age-weighted profit-sharing plans do have some potential disadvantages for the employer:

- If the key employees are younger than other employees, they will not receive as large a proportion of employer contributions;
- Administrative costs are higher because of actuarial calculations; and
- It is more difficult to explain the plan to employees.

401(K) PLANS

Internal Revenue Code Section 401(k) retirement savings programs allow employees to contribute on their own behalf, on a pre-tax basis, with the benefit of tax-deferred compounding similar to traditional IRAs, pension, and profit-sharing plans. The maximum allowable pre-tax contribution for employees is $18,000 for 2016; employees age 50 and over may be able to contribute an additional $6,000 via the "catch-up deferral." For physicians to be able to contribute the maximum allowable amount to their 401(k) plans, there generally must be participation from the lower-compensated employees in order to ensure that the plan is not discriminatory.

A traditional 401(k) plan is subject to two nondiscrimination tests: the actual deferral percentage (ADP) test for employee elective deferrals, and the actual contribution percentage (ACP) test for matching contributions. Now as an alternative, an employer may adopt a "safe harbor" 401(k) plan, which is not subject to nondiscrimination testing.

Under current tax law, there are two safe harbor alternatives to the ADP test. In the first, the employer makes a non-elective contribution of 3% to each eligible highly compensated and non-highly compensated employee. The other alternative offers the employer the opportunity to make matching contributions of 100% of non-highly compensated employee elective contributions up to 3% of pay, and 50% of non-highly compensated employee additional elective contributions up to 5% of pay. All matches and non-elective contributions made to satisfy the safe harbor must be immediately vested. In addition, the employer must notify employees within a reasonable period of time prior to the plan year, of their rights and obligations under the safe harbor arrangement.

By meeting the above criteria, many highly compensated owner/physicians will find they can actually accrue a greater benefit for themselves. With the objective of most qualified retirement plans being tax-advantaged growth for future income needs, obviously the greater amount allowed to be invested annually can make a dramatic difference down the road. Often acting as contribution limitations, guidelines are in place to ensure there is not a great disparity of contributions, with highly compensated key employees receiving the lion's share. The "safe harbor" alternative to the traditional 401(k) plan will enable many physicians to accrue a greater retirement benefit while still conforming to IRS guidelines. Based on the history of prior employee participation, the "safe harbor plan" may prove to be a viable alternative for those wanting to maximize their retirement planning options.

Roth 401(k)

Roth IRAs have become an extremely popular option for those who prefer the unique advantage of being able to withdraw funds during their retirement years on a tax- free basis, as opposed to traditional IRAs where withdrawals are taxed as ordinary income. The only real downside to Roth IRAs is that contributions are made on an after- tax basis and are not tax deductible like a traditional IRA. Unfortunately, most physicians have not been able to utilize Roth IRAs due to their relatively high income levels. The Roth IRA eligibility phase out for 2016 is between $116,000 and $131,000 for single filers and $183,000 to $193,000 for married taxpayers filing a joint tax return. However, as of January 1, 2006, highly compensated individuals who were unable to contribute to Roth IRAs, as well as younger workers expecting to be in higher tax brackets during their retirement years, are able to take advantage of a unique tax-advantaged savings plan called the "Roth 401(k)."

As its name implies, the Roth 401(k) incorporates elements of both traditional 401(k) plans and Roth IRAs. The Economic Growth and Tax Relief Reconciliation Act (EGTRRA) of 2001 allowed workers to make greatly expanded Roth IRA contributions, without any income restrictions impacting eligibility. Contributions for Roth IRAs in 2016 are limited to a maximum of $5,500 for taxpayers under age 50, and $6,500 for those 50 and older. The Roth 401(k) maximum contribution level, on the other hand, enables workers under age 50 to contribute up to $18,000, while workers age 50 and older will be able to contribute as much as $24,000. At that point, an employee currently contributing to a traditional 401(k) plan would have the option of simply having their contributions diverted to a Roth version of the plan. That election would impact the amount of take home salary since the contributions will be made on an after-tax basis, as opposed to pre-tax contributions made into a traditional 401(k) plan.

While all of this appears quite straightforward, there are a few nuances to consider prior to making the switch. First, matching employer contributions still must be made and invested in the traditional 401(k) account, not the Roth 401(k) account. Even if the employee makes all of their contributions exclusively to a Roth 401(k) account, they would still owe tax on retirement withdrawals from funds contributed by the employer, which were made on a tax-deductible basis, as well as the earnings on those contributions. Secondly, workers should also be aware that the annual deferral limits apply to all 401(k) contributions, regardless of whether they are made on a pre-tax or after-tax basis. While employees are allowed to contribute to both types of 401(k) plans, contributions to the traditional plan may need to be reduced or discontinued to comply with the over limits.

Employees considering the Roth option should know that, like the traditional 401(k) but unlike the Roth IRA, they will be required to begin mandatory minimum distributions by April 1st of the year following attainment of age 70 ½. This may be avoided by rolling over the Roth 401(k) to a Roth IRA, thus avoiding the minimum distribution rules.

403(b) Plans

The 403(b) is a tax-deferred retirement plan, similar to the 401(k) plan, but available only to employees of public educational institutions and some non-profit (tax-exempt) organizations.

Unlike the 401(k), the 403(b) is not required to abide by the Employee Retirement Income Security Act (ERISA) rules, even though many consider it a "qualified" plan. This is a blessing to the plan administrators, since ERISA requires plan administrators to monitor all levels of a 401(k) plan.

Like the 401(k) plans, 403(b) plans have the standard penalty-free distribution age of 59 ½, but with an exception: If the employee separates from services in the year turning 55 and is considered retired, there will be no early 10% withdrawal penalty.

A 403(b) plan is similar to a 401(k) plan in that the investment earnings grow tax-deferred until withdrawal, at which time they are taxed as ordinary income. The 403(b) plan may also include a 403(b) Roth provision allowing employee after-tax contributions. Employers are allowed to match the total contributions the employee makes into both plans, but will only be able to deposit matches into the traditional (non-Roth) 403(b) account.

As is the case with 401(k) plans, maximum allowable pre-tax contributions are $18,000 for 2016. Employees age 50 and over may also be able to contribute an additional $6,000 via the "catch-up deferral."

The greatest advantages of a 403(b) plan, as compared to the 401(k) plan, are for the plan administrators and the employees who decide to retire between ages 55 and 59. For more detailed information on 403(b) plans, visit the website www.403bwise.com.

457 Plans

The 457 plan is a tax-advantaged defined contribution retirement plan available only for government and non-church tax-exempt organizations. The plan is similar to the 401(k) and 403(b) plans with a few differences.

Unlike the 401(k), there is no 10% tax penalty for withdrawals before age 59 ½, though federal income taxes do apply. Employees can begin distributions of funds at any age, once they are retired, without any consequences. Employees can also withdraw funds if the account value does not exceed $5,000 and there have been no contributions to the plan for two years.

Another difference between the plans is that 457 plan contributions are not subject to the typical combined maximum contribution limitation. Employees can contribute the annual maximum amount of $18,000 to a 403(b), 401(k), or a combination of both to total $18,000, in addition to contributing the annual maximum amount of $18,000 to their 457 plan. Therefore, employees can contribute a total annual maximum amount of $36,000 a year by having a 403(b) or 401(k) in addition to a 457 plan. They can also contribute the catch-up contribution to the 403(b) or

401(k) and their 457 plan, if their 457 plan is a government plan, which would allow for an annual contribution of $48,000 for 2016. Non-governmental 457 plans do not provide the option to make a catch-up contribution. Please note that the maximum allowable contribution to a 401(k), 401(k) Roth, 403(b), and 403(b) Roth is a combined total of $18,000 for 2016.

The 457 plan also provides two types of catch-up provisions. The first is the catch-up contribution of $6,000 if age 50 and older. The second is available only to 457 plans and cannot be used with the first catch-up provision. The three-year 457 catch-up rule states that the employee can contribute another annual maximum contribution to his or her 457 account, as long as the employee is within three years of retirement. If an employee is at least 50 years old, within three years of retiring, and is participating in both a 403(b) and 457 plan, he or she will be able to contribute a total of $60,000 for 2016 ($24,000 for 403(b) plan, $18,000 for 457 plan and another $18,000 contribution for one of the three-year catch-ups). This provision enables you to make up for contributions not deferred in previous years. You may catch-up for any year(s) since January 1, 1979, if you were eligible to contribute, but did not contribute the maximum allowable amount.

SIMPLE PLANS

The Small Business Job Protection Act of 1996 created a unique retirement plan called SIMPLE, an acronym for Savings Incentive Match Plan for Employee. SIMPLE replaces the salary-reduction version of the Simplified Employee Pension, also known as SARSEP. The SIMPLE allows small business owners to put aside money easily and inexpensively in tax-deferred accounts for themselves and their employees.

To take advantage of this new form of retirement savings, the business entity must have no more than 100 employees and cannot use any other retirement plan in the same year. Also, eligible employees must have earned at least $5,000 in any two previous years from the same employer and be likely to do so in the current year.

SIMPLEs are available in two forms: a SIMPLE individual retirement account and a SIMPLE 401(k). SIMPLE IRAs can be set up for each employee for a nominal fee at a bank, mutual fund company or brokerage firm. SIMPLE 401(k) plans are more expensive, mainly because of administrative costs.

SIMPLEs allow owners and employees to defer a percentage of their compensation, up to $12,500 a year for 2016, indexed for inflation, with a "catch-up" provision for workers age 50 and over, allowing an additional $3,000 to be contributed. Owners may contribute to employees' plans either by contributing a matching contribution of 100% of the first 3% of participating workers' annual compensation deferred, up to a maximum of $12,500, or by contributing 2% of compensation up to $5,300 in 2016, for all workers, whether or not they participate in the salary deferral portion of the plan. Because the SIMPLE is a newer form of retirement plan, many options must be considered before implementation. On the positive side, SIMPLEs require no discrimination testing (which requires a certain relation between the amount of compensation deferred by the group of participants included in the lower level of compensation and those in the higher level of compensation), employees need not participate for a business owner to defer up to $12,500 plus the 3% match per year.

The traditional 401(k) plan limits an employer's tax deferral by the amount employees put into the plan. In addition, the employer has no fiduciary responsibility for employee investments under the SIMPLE arrangement.

The physician who wants to save more for retirement and take a bigger deduction may find the maximum contribution confining. Other qualified plans allow an employer to deduct as much as 100% of his or her salary up to $53,000 per year. Also, since SIMPLE money is fully vested from the beginning, the plan provides little incentive for employee loyalty.

Table 11-1 summarizes many of the basic characteristics of qualified plan alternatives for non-academic, for-profit employers.

Table 11-2 outlines the differences in the plans offered exclusively to academic institutions and not-for-profit organizations.

WHAT PLAN OFFERS THE RIGHT FIT?

There are many factors to consider when evaluating the different types of retirement plans for a medical practice. Table 11-3 will help you evaluate the benefits of each and narrow the alternatives. Of course, consulting with retirement experts before making a final decision is critical.

The options for tax-advantaged savings for retirement are numerous. The key is to spend the time to determine the options available to you, and then formulate a plan to maximize contributions.

Table 11-1. Qualified Plans Compared

Feature	Defined Benefit Plans		
	All DB Plans	Money Purchase Pension	Profit S
Employer contributions deductible?	Yes	Yes	Yes
Employer contributions to participant currently taxable?	No	No	No
Earnings accumulate with income tax deferred?	Yes	Yes	Yes
Maximum annual employer contribution or deduction?	Determined by actuary	100% of compensation up to $53,000	100% of con up to $53,00
Employer contributions required?	Yes	Yes	No
Employer contribution is allocated:	N/A	As a percentage of total covered compensation. Integrated with Social Security.	As a percenta covered com Integrated w Security.
Employee contributions required?	No	No	No
Maximum participant benefits (for defined benefit plans) or allocations (for defined-contribution plans)	Lesser of 100% of compensation or $210,000 annually	Lesser of 25% of compensation or $53,000	Lesser of 25 pensation or
Investments can be self-directed by participants?	No	Yes	Yes
What plan participants are favored by the plan design?	Older, closer to retirement, highly compensated	Highly compensated	Highly comp
What will participants' account value at retirement depend on?	Formula of the plan, which can be calculated based on years before retirement, compensation, years of service	The amount of contributions The number of years until retirement Investment return	Frequency an of contributi Number of ye retirement Investment re
Who bears investment risk?	Employer	Employee	Employee

Source: Mary Jo Stvan, President, Merit Benefits, Oakbrook, IL

Defined Contribution Plans			
Age-Weighted Profit Sharing	**SIMPLE**	**401(k)**	**Roth 401(k)**
Yes	Yes	Yes	Yes
No	No	No	Yes
Yes	Yes	Yes	Yes
100% of compensation up to $53,000	100% match up to 3% of compensation or 2% of compensation of all eligible employees	Generally, an employer may provide contributions in the form of a matching percentage of employee deferral.	Generally, an employer may provide contributions in the form of a matching percentage of employee deferral. If so, such amounts are contributed to the employee's pre-tax account, not the Roth account.
No	Yes	No	No
Based on number of years before participant reaches retirement age.	Pro-rata by compensation.	Based on the matching policy in effect.	Based on the matching policy in effect.
No	No	No	No
Lesser of 25% of compensation or $53,000	Lesser of 100% of compensation or $12,500	Lesser of a combined contribution (aggregated with other plans) of $18,000/$24,000 if under/over age 50 or 100% of compensation	Lesser of a combined contribution (aggregated with other plans) of $18,000/$24,000 if under/over age 50 or 100% of compensation
Yes	Yes	Yes	Yes
Older, closer to retirement, highly compensated	Younger	Younger	Younger
Frequency and amount of contributions Number of years until retirement Investment return	Frequency and amount of contributions Number of years until retirement Investment return	Frequency and amount of contributions Number of years until retirement Investment return	Frequency and amount of contributions Number of years until retirement Investment return
Employee	Employee	Employee	Employee

Table 11-2. Plans Offered by Academic Institutions

Description	403(b)	4C
Available for	Public education organizations and non-profit employers	Any employer; cor
Employee Maximum Annual Contributions (Deferral)	A combined contribution (aggregated with other plans) of Also available is the catch-up contribution of $6,000 for t inflation each year.	
Employer Max. Annual Contribution (Deferral)	Employer matches or other employer contributions, $53,000 or 100% of compensation (whichever is less).	Employer matches compensation (wh plan not the Roth
Employee Contributions Deductible?	Yes	Yes
Taxes	Contributions are taxed upon distribution.	
Loan Provisions	Loans available for 403(b) and 401(k) plans but not availa plans.	
Distributions	Age 59½ or older (55 if retired and other provisions may apply) are not subject to penalty, but are subject to federal taxes. Early distributions 10% penalty and 20% withheld for federal taxes All withdrawals are subject to federal taxes.	Age 59½ or older a penalty, but are su taxes. Early distrib 10% penalty and 2 for federal taxes.
Minimum Required Distribution	Must begin withdrawing required distribution no later tha	
Tax Qualified Rollover	Allowable to an IRA, Rollover IRA, 401(k), and 403(b).	

Source: MEDIQUS Asset Advisors, Inc., Chicago, IL

	401(k) Roth	Deferred Compensation (457)
ate sectors		Governmental and certain non-governmental (non-profit) employers
00% of compensation (whichever is less). of age and older. Amounts are adjusted for		A contribution (not aggregated with other plans) of $18,000 or 100% of compensation (whichever is less). Also available is the catch-up of $6,000 for those 50 years of age and older, but may not use while using the 457 three-year catch-up provision (see 457 write-up). Amounts are adjusted for inflation each year.
loyer contributions, $53,000 or 100% of). Matches for Roth are placed in the 401(k)		Employer matches or other employer contributions, $53,000 or 100% of compensation (whichever is less).
	No	Yes
	Contributions are initially taxed, but earnings are tax-free upon distribution.	Contributions are taxed upon distribution.
)(7)	Loans not available for plan.	Loans available for plan.
ct to al a eld	Age 59½ or older with a five-year waiting period, plan is not subject to penalty, but federal taxes do apply. Early distributions incur a 10% penalty and 20% is withheld for federal taxes.	Available after service ends at any age without penalty. While in service, if plan has less than $5,000 and has been inactive for two years, employee may take it as a de minims distribution. Federal taxes do apply.
owing the year in which age 70½ is reached.		
	Allowable to a Roth IRA or Roth 401(k).	Able to rollover into IRA, 401(k) and 403(b) plans. ONLY non-governmental 457 plan can be rolled into some type of 457 plan or an IRA once service is finished.

Table 11-3. Evaluating Retirement Plans

Plan Type	If you need flexibility in making deposits	If you would be the oldest, most highly compensated, or closest to retirement of all participants	If you would be able to afford contributions that would exceed 25% of participant compensation
Defined Benefit	unlikely to consider	definitely consider	definitely consider
Money Purchase Pension Plan	may consider	consider	no impact
Profit Sharing	definitely consider	unlikely to consider	consider
Age-Weighted Profit Sharing	definitely consider	definitely consider	consider
SIMPLE Plan	definitely consider	unlikely to consider	unlikely to consider

CHAPTER 12

Managing the Unwanted: Malpractice, Disability, and Impairment

Peter S. Moskowitz, MD, and Thomas Shapira, Esq.

PHYSICIANS ARE NOT WELL-PREPARED FOR unexpected problems such as malpractice, disability, and impairment, yet they are a harsh reality for many. The curriculum of most medical schools and the post-graduate training of interns, residents and fellows fails to prepare physicians-in-training to navigate these troubled waters. We hope to provide you with a general understanding of how to anticipate, avoid, and manage yourself and your medical career should any of these disasters befall you or a professional colleague.

MEDICAL MALPRACTICE

Medical malpractice is defined as any act or omission by a physician during treatment of a patient that deviates from accepted norms of practice in the medical community and causes an injury to the patient. Medical malpractice is a specific subset of tort law that deals with professional negligence.

Common Settings, Causes, and Outcomes

A JAMA study published in 2011 reported that 48% of paid malpractice claims were for events in in-patient settings, 43% in out-patient settings, and 9% in both.[1] A recent extensive review of this subject revealed that 70% of paid claims were in office-based solo practice and 64% were in single-specialty groups.[1] Ownership may play a role in the higher risk in solo practices and single-specialty groups.

Lawsuits in the out-patient setting are more likely to be due to diagnostic issues, such as misdiagnosis, and in the in-patient setting from surgical errors, such as leaving surgical instruments in the body.[1]

Other common circumstances leading to lawsuits include:

- Injuries or death during surgery;
- Postoperative infection;

- Late diagnosis or misdiagnosis of cancer;
- Misdiagnosed cardiac emergency;
- Late or misdiagnosis of birth defects or fetal death;
- Negligence during childbirth and childbirth injuries;
- In-hospital infections;
- Falls in hospital room; and
- Medication errors.

Despite the large number of malpractice proceedings initiated against physicians, only about one-third to one-half of those cases ever reach the trial phase. Of the other two-thirds of cases that do not go to trial, approximately three-fourths are eventually dropped by the plaintiff for a variety of reasons, the most common being that the plaintiff and legal team decide they do not have a strong case. Fewer than 10% of claims are ever settled by the court. The remaining cases are settled out of court by negotiation between the physician's malpractice legal team, the physician's malpractice insurer, and the plaintiff and his or her legal team.[2]

Of those relatively few cases that reach the trial phase, the majority are resolved in favor of the physician. While that is good news, even a successful trial result does not compensate the physician for the many hours of preparation time, worry, lost sleep, and time away from clinical practice, during the many months of proceedings.

Of those cases that are decided against the physician, the average malpractice settlement in the United States in the in-patient setting is $363,000, and $290,000 in the out-patient setting.[2,3] Of course, settlement amounts can vary from a few thousand dollars to multi-million dollar settlements, depending on the circumstances.

Regardless how a medical malpractice suit is resolved, a lawsuit has a negative impact on all physicians.

The Impact of Medical Malpractice on the Physician

Without doubt, there is nothing more impactful and stressful for a physician than being sued for malpractice. Because part of physicians' personality profile includes being excessively responsible, prone to perfectionism, and wanting to please others, a malpractice suit implies that a physician's best efforts have failed. That implication becomes internalized as "I am a failure as a physician."

Whether the accusations in the suit are true or not, the internal dialogue in the physician's mind too often leads to obsession over the details, how things might have been done differently, fear about the potential loss of respect from colleagues and the public, fear of economic loss, and the shame of not being perceived as perfect. There is an inevitable loss of self-esteem and a loss of self-confidence. Feelings of guilt and shame are almost always present whether conscious or unconscious and whether justified by the facts of the case or not.

The end result is a change in mood. Anxiety and depression are common manifestations of malpractice stress. If not dealt with effectively, the constellation of emotional challenges eventually can result in the degradation of the physician's physical and emotional health.

MANAGING STRESS DURING LITIGATION

The best legal defense is of little consolation if a physician is unable to take good care of himself or herself during this highly stressful time. Below, we offer our detailed approach to managing stress and improving self-care during litigation—an approach we hope you will never have to initiate during your professional career.

When the Summons Arrives

After you have recovered from the initial shock of receiving a summons, the most appropriate first step is to contact your insurance carrier to report the claim. Confirm your coverage as soon as possible. If your carrier is obligated to defend you, it will assign counsel of its choosing; however, if you have counsel that you prefer, you should request such counsel be assigned to your case. Your preferred counsel might not be on the carrier's "approved" list, so you may need to push your carrier to approve your counsel or identify other acceptable counsel off the "approved" list. Make a measured decision. If necessary, consult with colleagues or physician friends for their recommendation of a malpractice defense attorney.

Once a decision has been made regarding the best malpractice defense attorney to represent you, make an appointment to begin the preparation of your defense. This will help relieve your anxiety about the case and give you confidence that you are moving in the right direction to defend yourself.

Working with Your Legal Team

Your initial meetings with your defense attorney and staff will clarify the legal process, including what you can expect to occur in the subsequent weeks and months and what you can do to help them defend you. As the defendant, you must provide your legal team with all documentation and information that pertains to your care of the plaintiff patient and copies of all of your clinical care notes, records, and your written retrospective comments about everything that led up to the filing of the lawsuit.

The best way to handle the fear and anxiety of a malpractice lawsuit is to educate yourself as fully as possible about the procedural details that are to follow and to study the medical details of the alleged malpractice action. Your preparation must be thorough so you will be a credible and knowledgeable defendant for your deposition and later for the trial if the case reaches a trial phase.

Read and learn about every aspect of your case. Let your attorney guide your study and help prepare you for your testimony at a deposition and at trial. Practice testifying with your attorney.

Prepare yourself with the same vigor, determination, and hard work that you would devote to preparing yourself for a board exam or recertification exam. The better prepared you are, the more self-confident and the less fearful you will be. Nothing is as important as good preparation to sustain you during the long, often frustrating and emotionally trying time that lies ahead.

Managing Litigation Stress

Patients in our society expect professional practice perfection and that is what physicians expect to provide. When accusations of medical malpractice arise, they immediately affect the physician's sense of well-being and self-confidence. Feelings of fear, failure, anxiety, and depression are common. Because defense attorneys typically advise physicians not to discuss their case with anyone other than the legal team, physicians are left to deal with these difficult thoughts and feelings in isolation. This exacerbates the stress.

Managing the stress of malpractice litigation must become the physician's primary responsibility, although it is a task for which physicians are not typically prepared. The basic elements of a litigation stress management program should include all of the following:

Participate in Regular Aerobic Exercise. Aerobic exercise is perhaps the single most-effective way to combat litigation stress. The endorphin response generated by exercise increases energy, elevates mood, and increases the overall sense of well-being.

While the proper amount and intensity of exercise necessary is a topic of debate among wellness experts, a program of 30 minutes of aerobic exercise (sufficient to elevate the heart rate and result in perspiration) done a minimum of four days a week works well for most adults. Weight training can be alternated with cardio training. When access to appropriate training facilities is difficult, rapid walking for 30 minutes, four days a week, is a satisfactory substitute as long as it elevates the resting heart rate and induces sweat.

Maintain a Healthy Diet and Body Weight. All physicians have a general knowledge of what constitutes healthy eating. A well-balanced diet that includes the daily recommendations for vitamins, minerals, water, protein, carbohydrates, and fat, and that maintains body weight within approved limits based on body mass and height, fulfills this recommendation. Published guidelines for body weight based on height or total body mass index are readily available. When in doubt, or when a physician has a particular problem losing weight to meet acceptable standards, consulting a dietician can be an excellent way to get support and confirm that one's diet is appropriate in both content and in portion size.

Avoid Stimulants and Depressants. In the high-speed, high-stress world in which we live, it is common for healthcare professionals to use caffeine to sustain energy and focus during the workday. The growth of coffee emporiums and the pervasive advertising of caffeinated beverages are testaments to this phenomenon. To a physician under the added stress of medical malpractice litigation, caffeinated drinks may induce mood swings that increase the physician's underlying anxiety and may interfere with normal sleep cycles, adding to the stress and distress.

In a similar vein, beverages or medications that act as depressants are dangerous at all times, but particularly so for physicians facing the stress of malpractice litigation. The most common of these depressants are alcohol and barbiturates. The abuse and dependency potential for both alcohol and barbiturates is significant, particularly for people who are vulnerable to their abuse, such as people living in high-stress environments, physicians included. Because physicians in litigation are more prone to depression, depressants may promote and/or magnify clinical depression.

Physicians experiencing high levels of stress from any cause should refrain from the use of stimulants or depressants.

Get Adequate Restful Sleep. Sufficient sleep is in short supply in physicians' lives to begin with. A doctor who has too much on his or her plate will give up sleep in order to gain more time.

Sleep experts generally recommend at least eight hours of sleep every night for adults, particularly during periods of stress. Anything less than eight hours of sleep a night begins to degrade health. Under conditions of chronic sleep deprivation, physicians can begin to experience decreased performance and alertness, memory and cognitive impairment, deteriorating relationships, increased risk of occupational injury, mood volatility, irritability, depression, loss of appetite or overeating, hypertension, and increased risk of stroke and heart attack.

Physicians involved in a lawsuit should make adequate sleep the highest priority for their health and defense.

Maintain Close Contact with Friends and Family. The need for love, support, physical touch, and emotional understanding are fundamental needs of all human beings. Those who are isolated and alone for any reason suffer terribly because they are not getting those basic human needs met.

Who better can love and support us than our nuclear families? For that reason, doctors in litigation should prioritize time spent with their families, closest

friends, and other loved ones. While it is not appropriate or advisable to discuss any of the details of a lawsuit with family or friends, it is OK to let them know that you are fighting a lawsuit, that you need their love, support, and encouragement more than ever. Surround yourself with loving family and friends and make good use of their support.

Develop and Utilize a Professional Support System. Doctors in litigation must develop and utilize a good support system. Part of your support system may be your immediate family and close friends, as indicated above, but you must maintain appropriate boundaries with family and friends.

Seek out trusted professional friends and colleagues, where appropriate. Mental health professionals, clergy, and career and life coaches are also suitable sources for your support system. They are duty-bound to maintain your confidentiality. They are also trained to provide emotional support to people at times of crisis.

Your legal team will obviously be the most important part of your support system. Choose them wisely and actively seek their support and input as you prepare yourself to do battle.

Educate Yourself About Your Case and Your Defense. Physicians in litigation are beset with many emotions; without a doubt, the most pervasive emotion is fear: fear of the unknown, fear of having one's professional reputation damaged or destroyed, fear of the economic consequences of losing a trial, fear of losing patients. The most potent insulator from fear is knowledge. Educate yourself about the details of your case and how to best defend yourself in court. Know what to expect and be prepared.

Prioritize Time for Fun. In the heat of a battle, no one is thinking about fun. Yet, fun is another one of the pillars of stress reduction. Put fun on your calendar, in your iPhone to-do list, and find a few minutes every day for fun alone, with friends, and with family members. If necessary, ask your friends and family members for suggestions for fun activities. Fun will clear your mind, open your heart, and help propel you into another day with some happiness.

The Risk of Additional Lawsuits

Studies have documented that once a physician has been served papers for malpractice, he or she is three times more likely to be accused a second time. There may be many reasons for this phenomenon, but one of them could be that the stress and distraction of a lawsuit may affect a physician's clinical decision making, judgment, and ability to focus.

This supports the importance of effective stress reduction once a malpractice action begins. Stress reduction will promote physical and mental health; improve the physician's ability to focus on work and not obsess about the unknown, and to maintain a hopeful, positive outlook.

Decreasing Your Personal Risk

While no one piece of knowledge or strategy can totally insulate a physician from the risk of litigation, certain practice priorities and professional behaviors have been shown to decrease the risk of medical errors that may result in litigation.

Maintaining effective communication with patients is one of the most important professional behaviors to reduce the risk of medical malpractice litigation. Physicians must strive to explain to patients the medical diagnosis, all treatment options available, the potential adverse effects of those treatment options, and the prognosis for full recovery. When treatment outcomes are suboptimal, it is important to discuss why the result has not been as expected, and what new treatment options are available.

Whether mistakes of commission or omission have been made, the physician should face up to them and discuss what happened with the patient. Although how to handle this situation is subject to controversy, discussing mistakes directly with the patient has been shown to reduce the likelihood that the patient will sue.

Another key to limiting liability exposure for a physician from professional malpractice as well as any other liability is to practice medicine in the context of an entity, such as a professional or medical corporation, limited liability company, professional limited liability company, or professional association. Such an entity can be used for a sole practitioner as well. A partnership (which does require at least one other owner) is not an entity that offers sufficient protection against liability in the context of a medical practice.

In most states, a physician's professional liability extends to the physician's personal assets, which cannot be shielded by formation of an entity. However, a properly formed entity can shield a physician against professional liability by another physician in the group, as well as against liability for claims other than professional liability. Such other liability includes a patient's personal injury, such as a slip and fall in the waiting area, a fall off an examination table, or employee claims for discrimination or sexual harassment.

A partner in a partnership is "jointly and severally" liable for all liabilities of the partnership regardless of his partnership share. "Joint and several" means that a creditor can pursue any one partner for the full amount of the liability, leaving that partner to try to get some contribution from his or her other partners. The partner's personal assets (e.g., house, car, etc.) can be seized to satisfy the liability.

Unlike a partnership, in an entity such as a corporation or limited liability company, an owner (e.g., shareholder, member) is liable only for his or her respective share of the assets of the entity. Yes, the owner could lose his or her entire investment in the practice, including all accounts receivable, but the physician can take comfort in the fact that his or her personal assets are not exposed. Assuming the physician is not the party who is alleged to have committed malpractice, the patient/plaintiff will sue the responsible physician as well as the physician group entity. The patient/plaintiff will not be able to successfully sue another physician in the group on an individual basis. Similarly, if the practice incurs any other liability, it is the entity and not an individual owner who will be responsible. Accordingly, creating an entity for the medical practice is an essential step in limiting liability.

While no one piece of knowledge or strategy can totally insulate a physician from the risk of litigation, certain practice priorities and professional behaviors have been shown to decrease the risk of medical errors that may result in litigation.

Maintaining effective communication with patients is one of the most important professional behaviors to reduce the risk of medical malpractice litigation. Physicians must strive to explain to patients the medical diagnosis, all treatment options available, the potential adverse effects of those treatment options, and the prognosis for full recovery. When treatment outcomes are suboptimal, it is important to discuss why the result has not been as expected, and what new treatment options are available.

Whether mistakes of commission or omission have been made, the physician should face up to them and discuss what happened with the patient. Although how to handle this situation is subject to controversy, discussing mistakes directly with the patient has been shown to reduce the likelihood that the patient will sue.

The Aftermath

Win or lose, you will feel some combination of relief, regret, shame, and anger in the end. Very likely you will also feel gratitude for those who helped and supported you through the complexities of the legal system. Find genuine, heart-felt ways to thank those who deserve your thanks. You will know immediately who they are.

The negative feelings—and there will always be negative feelings—will not go away overnight. Unrestrained, they have the potential to consume you and keep you mired in blackness, shielding you from happier times. Therefore, it is good to have a strategy for dealing with these negative emotions and memories.

If you work hard to recover, eventually you will heal and prosper again as a person and as a physician. Your self-confidence will return. Wiser now, you hopefully will again enjoy the practice of medicine. However, you will be more cautious and perhaps a bit more suspicious as a practitioner.

Strategies for Recovery

Recovering from the effects of a malpractice lawsuit can be challenging, regardless of the outcome of the case. The very fact that a patient accused you of malpractice is difficult for physicians to handle emotionally. We expect nothing short of perfection of ourselves. We may experience guilt, shame, anger, lingering self-doubt, and low self-esteem.

These emotions are sometimes difficult to manage alone. People I know who have recovered from traumatic malpractice experiences have utilized a variety of strategies to do so.

The simple and obvious things that can sustain physicians after a lawsuit include spending more time with family and friends, taking more time off for fun, hobbies, and travel. Balancing life and work is the best long-term strategy. Talking about the experience with a mental health professional may offer relief.

Finally, know that time heals all wounds.

THE DISABLED PHYSICIAN

A physician may be considered disabled by any illness, injury, or mental infirmity that compromises the physician's ability to manage direct patient care. Disability may be temporary or permanent.

Temporary disability, while disruptive to the doctor's practice and staff, has no long-lasting impact on most physicians and they return to practice. Today, most doctors maintain both short-term and long-term disability insurance that supports their income while disabled.

Permanent disability, on the other hand, is an unfortunate disaster affecting the physician's patient panel, the physician's colleagues and staff, and the physician's economic viability. Without appropriate disability insurance, the impact on the physician's life can be devastating.

Common Causes and Impact

Acute infectious diseases, cardiovascular disease, musculoskeletal trauma, neoplastic diseases, and mental health conditions are the most common causes of short- and long-term disability among physicians. Over the course of a physician's career, it is estimated that up to 10% of physicians will experience at least one episode of short-term disability during their practice years.

Short-term and long-term disability may have a profound emotional effect on physicians. Spending time in a hospital or at home recuperating from an acute illness or accident is a challenge for most physicians, who tend to believe that any time they are not being productive is wasted time.

Once the physician's short-term illness (fewer than 6 months) is responding and the physician is able to read and correspond with others, the stress of the illness or injury can typically be handled with the support of loved ones and the medical team in charge. The temporary loss of income while recuperating is most often covered by disability insurance provided in the workplace or medical practice.

Long-term disability (more than 6 months) is another matter. Long-term disability is often permanent and may imply the inability to practice medicine, at least without significant accommodation. Moreover, there frequently is a significant emotional impact of long-term or permanent disability. Such long-term disability requires an entirely new outlook on one's personal and professional life which most people are unprepared to deal with. Depression and anxiety are common. Seeking the help of mental health professionals is the best recommendation to assist physicians deal with their loss and learn to move ahead.

Re-entry to professional life after permanent disability often requires extensive career planning and new training or learning. Later in this chapter, we provide a career coaching perspective on how to begin the planning process for that new career.

How to Protect Yourself from Disability

There is no way to anticipate the onset of an infectious disease, neoplasm, or injury. That said, it makes sense for all physicians to practice what they preach in terms of maintaining general health and wellness. At a minimum, every physician regardless of age should have an annual physical exam by a personal physician other than themselves, and follow the health and wellness guidelines recommended by that physician.

The Special Case of the Aging Physician

We've known for decades that there is a progressive decline in both physical and cognitive function over time. Physicians are no exception to that general rule. Until recently, there were no guidelines with which to evaluate the performance of older physicians. For the most part, physicians were left alone to determine when the time was right for them to retire from active practice. Generally, this was not a problem, but occasionally, poorly functioning physicians were recognized only after recurrent errors in judgment or errors of commission that adversely affected patient care and safety.

In many cases, it is the observations of a physician's declining mental or physical skills by his or her colleagues that pushes some doctors to retire or to modify their clinical activity to more appropriately match their declining effectiveness. Sadly, many physicians are reluctant, even after observing the declining function of a colleague, to speak up and confront the poorly functioning physician face to face.

There is a growing movement to require mandatory physical and cognitive testing of physicians when they reach the age of 65 or 70, with the intent of securing patient safety, and of identifying those physicians whose cognitive function might compromise their ability to practice medicine effectively and safely.[4] Time will tell whether these attempts to impose specific functional standards for the performance of aging physicians will be successful and be upheld if challenged in the legal system.

Issues with Licensing Agencies and Medical Boards

Depending on the severity of a physician's disability, the state Medical Board may or may not be involved. Nonpsychotic emotional/mental disabilities such as major depression are most often successfully managed on an out-patient basis by a physician's personal mental health professional. Individual psychotherapy with or without psychoactive medication need not be reported to state licensing agencies.

Emotional/mental disorders that require in-patient treatment need to be reported to the state Physician Health Program. Once the physician is able to return to clinical practice and the treating mental health professional(s) do not believe that patient safety is at risk, the Physician Health Program can assist with the re-entry and continue to monitor the performance of the physician.

Physical disabilities do not usually exclude clinical practice, although the workplace may need suitable accommodation for a physician's unique physical challenges.

Physicians impaired by substance abuse and other forms of addiction also have problems with state and local monitoring agencies or committees. These are addressed separately in the section devoted to physician impairment later in this chapter.

Career Planning after Long-Term Disability

In most cases of short-term disability there is no need for career planning. However, a re-assessment of a physician's career trajectory may become necessary when his or her disability becomes long-term (more than one year) or permanent. This can best be done with help from others.

Seek Professional Career Planning Assistance. Long-term disability may permit a physician to continue practicing medicine but with various accommodations suitable to the disability. Work hours may need to be shortened, procedures/surgery may need to be modified or abandoned. Patients typically are understanding in these situations, making work pattern changes easier for the disabled physician.

When a physical or emotional disability translates to having to find an entirely new way to make a professional living, the impact on the physician and the time required to become acclimated to this new reality are very significant. In situations such as this, it is incumbent on the physician to seek the services of a professional career coach or career counselor familiar with medical careers and medical career transitions.

Initiate a Medical Career Transition. Although the process to find a new career is often circuitous and lengthy, there are some basic principles and self-understanding upon which a physician can begin to develop a career transition plan. A full description of the work necessary is beyond the scope of this book. That said, there are four basic pillars of information that help to support a platform from which you can begin your search for a new career.

1. **Your purpose.** This is the reason you believe you are here on this planet, what you want to focus your energy and time on, what gets you out of bed in the morning.
2. **Your motivated skills.** These are the skills that you are good at and love using. Chances are good that whatever you choose to do next, you will be happier if you are able to use your motivated skills in that new job. A career professional can help you identify your motivated skills.
3. **Your personality style.** Your personality helps determine how you respond to people, what kind of work setting you are most suited to, your unique challenges in the workplace, and what types of careers people with your profile are most suited to. The Myers Briggs Personality Inventory is the gold standard in determining your personality style. They inventory can be administered by career planning professionals or you can take it online.
4. **Your most important career values.** These values, unique to you, help to define factors that affect your career satisfaction. Being clear about the values that are always important to you in the workplace will help you evaluate the suitability of new careers under consideration and point to potential value conflicts and congruencies. A career value assessment can be done with your career professional.

Obtain New Training or Education. Transitioning medical professionals who elect new careers within or outside of clinical medicine often need to supplement their college and medical school education, training, and practice experience with new training or learning. In some instances, that may mean a new period of training within their current field of work, or perhaps a new fellowship within their current field. Less commonly, it may mean retraining in an entirely new clinical field within medicine.

Those seeking new non-clinical careers may decide to take new coursework to update their technical, writing, teaching, or computer literacy. Some will obtain certification training in new non-clinical areas such as information technology, healthcare administration, research administration, consulting to private industry or the government, teaching, high-tech medical instrumentation, computer programming, wellness coaching, lifestyle medicine, to name just a few popular fields in today's new world of opportunity for physicians.

Obtaining new training or education will take time and money, meaning the transition to a new career will take some time. That investment in oneself, regardless of the time it takes or the expense, will make all of the difference between a hastily conceived career change that is unsuccessful and a well-planned transition that includes education, skill building, and new life skills in preparation for success in today's increasingly complex technical society.

Stay Connected to Family, Friends, and Professional Networks. A good support system is crucial for successful career transitions. Your family, friends, and professional colleagues are terrific sources of support, and often useful in providing key networking resources. Since successful career transitions require courage and tenacity, your transitions will often be an inspiration to your loved ones and professional colleagues. It will also be a powerful lesson in resilience for your children.

A physician also needs the loving support of a spouse to pull off a successful career change. Working with a certified financial planner is often necessary to assure everyone that the proposed transition will be done in a way that will not financially destabilize the family.

You Can Do Almost Anything You Put Your Mind To

Ultimately, physicians can transition to just about any career they decide to pursue. Physicians have numerous transferrable skills, many of which they tend to overlook or not be aware of. Early in the career transition process, physicians say, "But my specialty is all that I know how to do! I can't see myself doing anything else!"

Working with a career transition professional who is familiar with medical careers and healthcare in general will be invaluable to the transitioning professional to overcome this negative belief. The career counselor/coach will provide support and encouragement, appropriate assessment tools, and most importantly, provide accountability to assure steady progress and help guide the transitioning physician to his or her new career goals.

THE IMPAIRED PHYSICIAN

A physician becomes impaired by any condition or influence that negatively affects his or her judgment, reasoning, or ethical behavior. The impairment can be temporary, long-term, or permanent.

The most common cause of physician impairment is abuse of mood-altering substances. Process addictions such as gambling, overeating, sexual addiction, and addictive shopping are far less common, and typically do not result in clinical practice impairment. Alcohol abuse/dependency is the most common cause of physician impairment. Abuse or dependence on prescription drugs, narcotics, and other painkillers is also more common among physicians. Alcohol is reported to be the most common drug of abuse among physicians (50%), followed by opioids (36%), stimulants (8%), and other substances (6%).[5,6]

Signs of Impairment

A patient or co-worker notes the smell of alcohol on a physician's breath in the workplace, during ordinary working hours. Such an observation warrants immediate, mandatory confrontation with a demand that the physician submit to immediate breath and/or urine screening for alcohol or other banned substances. Refusal to do so should be grounds for disciplinary action up to and including termination of employment and partnership.[7,8]

Additional warning signs may include chronic patterns of arriving late to work on Monday mornings; chronic tardiness in general; recurrent unexplained absences from the workplace during ordinary hours; failure to respond to pages or phone calls on emergency call duty; multiple clinical errors of omission or commission; multiple complaints about a physician's behavior by patients, families, and staff; and multiple malpractice claims against a physician over a relatively short period of time.

A physician impaired by alcohol or drugs is often emotionally unstable, irritable, defensive, and may show signs of depression and/or anxiety. Poor sleep and erratic eating patterns typically promote this emotional lability. Excessive amounts of coffee and other caffeine-containing substances may be consumed in an effort to compensate for the depressant effects of alcohol and some drugs. Chronic, secret consumption of barbiturates may be used to mask or modify the highs of methamphetamine and/or cocaine abuse.

Disability due to mental health issues occurs in physicians in higher incidence than in the general population. It has been said that as many as 10% of practicing physicians in the United States suffer from a classifiable Axis 1 or Axis 2 disorder.[7,8] The most common of these include major (unipolar) depression, bipolar depression, anxiety, and various personality disorders.

The association of substance abuse or dependency with major mental health disorders such as unipolar/bipolar depression is noteworthy. While the physician's behavior pattern may be the presenting feature, underlying and unrecognized substance abuse or dependency should be excluded by appropriate history and testing.

If Physician Impairment Is Suspected

For patient safety and the safety of the impaired physician, action should be taken after any initial "sentinel" event reported by patients, families, or co-workers. Impaired physicians threaten patient safety, commit more errors, and have a much higher incidence of malpractice litigation and more driving-under-the-influence convictions. The latter should also be considered a "sentinel event" to be investigated regarding possible chronic drug/alcohol dependency.

Impaired physicians are also three times more likely to commit suicide than non-impaired physicians—a tragedy that can often be prevented by appropriate recognition of and intervention in a physician's chemical dependency.[9]

The spouse or family members of a physician are often the first to suspect or observe a physician's pattern of excessive drinking or drug use. Because alcoholism tends to follow familiar patterns and be associated with shame and co-dependency, family members are often reluctant to confront the physician directly or to report the behavior to appropriate authorities. They understandably fear retribution and/or legal and professional practice consequences that may affect the physician. A conspiracy of silence and secrecy thus develops that shields the impaired physician until some unavoidable, often tragic mistake uncovers the truth.

Evidence of substance abuse may be recognized by physician peers but go unreported for some of the same reasons mentioned above for family members. By not confronting the situation, those who are reluctant to take action increase the risk of a tragic or fatal outcome for a patient, or for the physician in question.

Action(s) by Medical Executive Committees or Chiefs-of-Staff.

Evidence presented to the chief-of-staff or to the medical executive committee of a medical facility warrants confidential referral to the Physician Well-Being

Committee of that institution, if one exists. It is the duty of the Physician Well-Being Committee to interview the physician, review the facts and evidence, and make a determination as to whether there is reason to believe that the physician may be abusing or be dependent on mood-altering substances, or have a significant mental health disorder.

The committee has the power to engage the physician in a confidential, binding contract to ensure an appropriate referral(s) to an addiction specialist and/or a psychiatric specialist be made to establish a diagnosis, assess the physician's suitability to practice, and determine whether additional treatment for chemical dependency or a treatable Axis 1 or 2 disorder or major depression may be indicated to stabilize the physician's condition.

Action(s) by State Medical Boards

Nearly all state medical boards have special confidential Physician Health Programs that are charged with the investigation, contracting, treatment recommendations, post-treatment follow-up, and recovery surveillance. In those states in which there is no Physician Health Program, the state Medical Board performs these duties.

Specific details regarding the Physician Health Program (PHP) in your state can be found on the website for the state Medical Board. In all cases, the intent is that physicians are treated with sensitivity and respect. The PHP helps the physician get appropriate treatment for his or her addiction. Following treatment, PHP follow-up is performed to determine when and under what conditions the physician can return to clinical practice.

Rehabilitation and Recovery

Once a diagnosis of chemical dependency or major psychiatric illness is established, the healthcare institution where the physician practices, through its Well-Being of Physicians Committee, can help connect the physician to appropriate treatment. The work of the committee is confidential; however, a diagnosis of chemical dependency/addiction or a major psychiatric disorder may have to be reported to the state Medical Board, by law, in some states.

The Well-Being of Physicians Committee then monitors the involved physician over time, receives reports from treating physicians/recovery treatment programs, assists and supports the physician with follow-up care after discharge from in-patient care, and assists with re-entry to practice.

In-Patient Treatment Programs. The majority of physicians referred for treatment because of substance abuse disorders require in-patient care, typically 30 to 60 days in length. Physicians require longer primary treatment because they are held to a higher standard of treatment success than other non-healthcare professionals and the lay public.

The initial phase of treatment may have to include monitored detoxification of a week or more. All mood-altering substances must be out of the system before accurate psychological assessment, treatment planning, and recovery education can be performed.

It is customary that the in-patient treatment includes individual and group psychotherapy, regular attendance at 12-Step meetings, initial written work on The 12 Steps of Recovery, and education about addiction and recovery strategies. When clinically appropriate, additional treatment modalities may include physical therapy, occupational therapy, and dietary/nutrition consultation.

After traditional in-patient treatment, some patients require additional, less-intense treatment. For those patients, discharge to a sober living environment or halfway house for an additional period of time may be indicated before the physician is judged to be ready to re-enter clinical practice.

While in a sober living environment, patients will have several hours a day of group meetings, individual or group psychotherapy, and planning for re-entry. At other times of the day the patient may be engaged in part-time work, reading/learning, physical exercise, and spiritual activities including prayer, meditation, and 12-Step work.

Out-Patient Treatment Programs. Some physicians who need intensive treatment but who are emotionally stable and do not need detoxification may be suitable for intensive out-patient therapy to enter recovery. Under the supervision of an addiction psychiatrist and a physician boarded in addiction medicine, the physician may benefit from out-patient psychotherapy several times a week, attendance at 12-Step meetings, 12-Step sponsorship, appropriate medical treatment of depression or anxiety, steps to improve physical health and fitness, and random urine screening.

Support meetings specifically for recovering physicians, if available, are great sources of strength, and good resources for finding 12-Step sponsors. Physicians tend to do better with sponsors who themselves are recovering physicians.

Aftercare. A well-planned aftercare program is established for the patient to follow after release from the sober living environment. Such plans typically include ongoing psychotherapy in the physician's community, 12-Step recovery meeting attendance, a 12-Step sponsor in the patient's community, slow re-integration into clinical practice, and frequent monitoring that often includes unscheduled, random urine testing to document satisfactory progress in recovery.

In many states, periodic written documentation of satisfactory progress in recovery must be reported to the state Medical Board or the PHP for up to several years before the physician's license to practice medicine is fully restored without restrictions.

For a physician to sustain recovery for the remainder of his or her practicing years, he or she must make a long-term commitment to attending 12-Step meetings, working with a sponsor or a physician's recovery support group, and scrupulously avoiding situations and conditions that in the past triggered acting out behaviors.

The Importance of Work–Life Balance to Recovery

Of all recovery behaviors, perhaps the most important is to maintain work-life balance. Carnes has previously shown that the loss of consistent work-life balance is an early and accurate predictor of addiction relapse.[10] For physicians who are data-driven in their clinical decision making, a useful data-driven way to assess and monitor one's own work–life balance has been provided by Carnes. His Personal Craziness Index[10] is a simple and meaningful way to continuously monitor balance. The index is an excellent way for any physician, even those not in addiction recovery, to monitor their own work-life balance.

Support of Family and Loved Ones

Connection to others in recovery and the love and support of loved ones and family members are other important cornerstones of a solid recovery program. Connection to other recovering physicians is also key. That connection can be secured by attending 12-Step meetings and physicians-in-recovery group meetings, and working with a sponsor who is a recovering physician.

Maintaining the support of family and loved ones may seem obvious, however many physicians must work hard to rebuild trust in their intimate family relationships in order to earn that support. All too often, loved ones and family members have suffered difficult and painful consequences of the acting out behavior of the addicted physician prior to treatment and recovery.

Therefore, recovery behaviors, in addition to maintenance of sobriety and good self-care, must include making amends to those who have been damaged by the behavior of the addicted physician when appropriate, and focusing on rigorous honesty in all aspects of the physician's life and professional career.

Recidivism

Physicians have remarkable abstinence rates after completing an addiction/rehabilitation program compared with the general population. Abstinence rates are between 74% and 90%.5 These high rates could be due to motivation to maintain licensure and to continue professional practice, as well as the extensive treatment and long-term monitoring that are required of recovering physicians.

However, there is also a disturbing rate of recidivism for addicted physicians. The Washington State Physician's Health Program reviewed its experience with healthcare professionals during a 10-year period and found that 25% had at least one relapse and noted apparent contributing or confounding factors.[11] Relapse risk was increased by a family history of a substance use disorder, by a coexisting psychiatric illness (dual diagnosis), and a history of opioid addiction. When all three of these factors are present, there is a 13-fold increased risk of relapse.9

Because of the risk of suicide or overdose occurring during relapse, especially in those with a history of opioid addiction, addiction treatment and monitoring programs must account for these factors when treatment plans are being developed and when physicians are being counseled about returning to practice.

REFERENCES

1. Peckham C. Malpractice and medicine: who gets sued and why? *Medscape*. 2015, Dec 08.
2. Jena AB, Chandra A, Lakdawalla D, Seabury S. Outcomes of medical malpractice litigation against US physicians. *Arch Int Med*. 2012; 172(11):892–894.
3. Peters PG. Twenty years of evidence on the outcomes of malpractice claims. *Clin Orthop Relat Res*. 2009 Feb;467(2):352–357.
4. Moutier CY, Bazzo DE, Norcross WA. Approaching the issue of the aging physician population (data from the Coalition for Physician Enhancement Conference). *Journal of Medical Regulation*. 2013;99:10–18.
5. Berge KH, Seppala MD, and Schipper AM. Chemical dependency and the physician. *Mayo Clin. Proc.* 2009 Jul;84(7):625–631.
6. McClelland At, Skipper GS, Campbell M, DuPont RL. Five year outcomes in a cohort study of physicians treated for substance disorders in the United States. *BMJ*. 2008 Nov4:337:2038.
7. Rothstein L. Impaired physicians and the ADA. *JAMA*. 2015;313(22):2219–2220.
8. Baldisseri MR. Impaired healthcare professional. *Crit Care Med*. 2007;35(2 Suppl):S106-S116.
9. Menk EJ, Baumgarten RK, Kingsley CP, et. al. Success of re-entry into anesthesia training programs by residents with a history of substance abuse. *JAMA*. 1990;263(22):3060–3062.
10. Carnes P. *A gentle path through the twelve steps: The classic guide for all people in the process of recovery*. Center City, MN: Hazelden Press; 2012.
11. Domino KB, Hornbein TF, Polissar N, et. al. Risk factors for relapse in healthcare professionals with substance abuse disorders. *JAMA*. 2005;293(12):1453–1460.

The Late-Career Physician

CHAPTER 13

Getting Serious About Retirement

Peter S. Moskowitz, MD, and Neil H. Baum, MD

"More retirements fail for non-financial reasons than for financial reasons."

MK STEIN, *The Prosperous Guide to the New Retirement*

ONE OF THE MOST IMPORTANT DECISIONS a physician makes is when and how to leave the practice of medicine. Being prepared for retirement makes this critical decision—and the transition to retirement—easier.

Just a few decades ago, physicians worked until the day they died or were physically unable to practice anymore. Today, many physicians begin thinking about their retirement from medicine well before they are ready to hang up their stethoscopes. Starting the planning process in the early stage of practice greatly enhances your chances of success when your retirement date rolls around.

PROTIRING VS RETIRING

Retirement means different things to different people. In fact, a quick check in the Practical Standard Dictionary shows six definitions for retirement:

1. To pay up, withdraw from circulation
2. To separate or withdraw
3. To go into privacy or seclusion
4. To withdraw from service or public life
5. To draw back, go away
6. To sink out of sight

We are willing to bet none of these phrases describes your vision of retirement. The Boomer generation is re-writing the rules for living. Many are working productively into their 70s and 80s. Others leave their lifetime careers in their 60s to work in new areas of interest, start new businesses of their own, volunteer their skills in any one of a number of ways, stay physically active and healthy, and enjoy life more than at any other time in their lives.

Today, an increasing number of people are opting to protire—to retire from their current job and pursue something else that gives their lives meaning. Protirement means to proactively plan for our later life and career. Ideally, protirement begins early in one's career and involves one's partner or spouse in the planning process.

As a part of your protirement plan, we recommend that you consult a certified financial planner to help you evaluate the many financial challenges of moving from a steady, predictable working income to a retirement income that may be somewhat lower or less predictable than what you are accustomed to.

With your spouse or partner, you will need to develop a vision of what your lifestyle in retirement will look like and project the cost of that lifestyle forward to the year you plan to leave your present career. Your protirement plan should take into consideration the needs and goals of spouses/partners. As you begin to develop your individual visions for protirement, it is not unusual for you to discover some differences in priorities for your time, your money, or how you intend to have fun or keep busy. When these differences arise, seek win-win strategies. In other words, both partners may have to compromise a bit so that you reach negotiated solutions that are acceptable to both of you, without either partner feeling they have been forced to surrender, or given in too much to the other.

The secret to success is revisiting your protirement plan annually. As you get older, your family grows, your physical health changes, and your nest egg for retirement grows, so you may want to revise your protirement plan to reflect the new realities in your life.

GENERAL RECOMMENDATIONS FOR YOUR PROTIREMENT PLAN

To protire means to retire from medicine to something else that gives your life meaning and gives you a sense of contribution to society. The happiest and best-adjusted physicians in retirement are those who have left medicine in order to do something that they are interested in and passionate about.

In defining what that "something else" might be, clarify and consider your own unique skills, interests, and passions. It you don't know what your own skills, interests, and passions are, you may benefit from a few sessions with a certified career counselor or career coach.

Volunteering your time prior to retirement is a good way to explore possibilities for your protirement. Physicians often are not aware of their own unique skills and have no idea what other kinds of work might be feasible and stimulating. One of the easiest and most valuable ways to obtain that knowledge is by volunteering.

Begin by making a list of any work or careers you have considered doing and a list of all of the things you find interesting. Now find out if there are any volunteer opportunities in any of these areas. Volunteer on your days off, on weekends, or on vacation time.

You won't regret the time you devote to volunteering prior to retirement and it may well inform what you choose to do during retirement. Some of the areas might require training or learning, but when you are retired, you will have the time and resources for that training or learning.

Work with a financial planning professional long before your retirement date. Throughout this book, the authors emphasize ways in which the guidance of certified financial planners and estate planning professionals can help physicians navigate the complexities of their practice lives. Almost all practicing physicians are too engaged in patient care and their own families to do a good job of managing their own retirement assets. Furthermore, protirement will involve complex calculations regarding income needs and income streams in retirement. A team of professional financial advisors can take the stress and worry out of setting up your retirement and protirement plans and help bring them to fruition.

Make sure you have a well-considered, written financial plan for retirement prepared by your certified financial planner. Your plan must consider in great detail the lifestyle you and your spouse/partner envision for your 30+ years of retirement and protirement and the annual cost of that lifestyle in today's dollars. Then adjust it for inflation over the years you are likely to live after retirement. Failure to plan in this way is planning to fail in retirement.

Create an income plan for retirement that will cover your lifestyle expenses until age 90. Physicians should plan to have an adequate income stream through age 90. Not all of us will be lucky to live to age 90, but Americans are more vigorous and healthy, and live much longer than in prior decades. After all, you should have been walking your talk and taking good care of yourself, your health needs, and your wellness.

Income stream calculations are complex and should be done in conjunction with your certified financial planner. Just as your overall retirement plan should be in writing, so should your income stream plan. Most conservative financial planners recommend that you should plan your lifestyle in retirement to cost no more than 4% annual withdrawal from your retirement assets. Structured in this way, you should not outlive your retirement assets.

Don't be overly conservative with the investments in your retirement plan. Putting all of your money into safe bets such as bonds and CDs, thinking it will protect you from major market downturns, will not be a successful strategy long-term. Remember that bonds and CDs will not beat inflation long-term, and it is likely you will need your money for another 30 years or longer. Be sure your portfolio is well-diversified and that at least 40% of your total retirement assets are in well-diversified securities.

Don't plan on Social Security being a major income source in retirement. For decades, workers have had peace of mind knowing that they could depend on their monthly Social Security stipend to help support themselves in retirement. Initially, many people were able to live off of their monthly Social Security payment. Over the decades, inflation and the cost of living have eroded the purchasing power of the dollar. The majority of physicians live in urban and suburban locations where the cost of living is highest. The end result is that Social Security payments comprise less than 50% of most physicians' monthly income requirements in retirement; for many it is even lower. Furthermore, the long-term survival of the entire Social Security system is in question, and to a large extent shrouded by the whims of the American political system.

Be sure to consult your financial planner as you near the age for Social Security eligibility. While you may need to start receiving Social Security payments at age 62, the longer you can defer payments the larger your monthly payments will be, up to age 70. In general, your payments increase by approximately 8% for each year you defer between age 66 and 70. Also discuss with your financial planner when your spouse should begin taking Social Security payments. In many instances, there is a clear advantage for the spouse of a physician to defer payments.

The bottom line: As you develop your retirement income plan, you would be prudent to assume that your monthly Social Security projected payment may not be secure. The safest approach: Plan your retirement finances with the assumption that Social Security may cease to exist within the next decade. If it does survive, that will be icing on your retirement cake.

Assume you will need 80% to 100% of your current income in retirement. We often read articles by financial planners saying that one should plan on retirement expenses to be no more than 75% to 80% of your maximum pre-retirement income. That assumption was predicated on the fact that in retirement, one's federal income tax rate decreases and one's lifestyle expenses tend to gradually diminish the older we get.

We live in a much different world today. Tax rates often fluctuate with the affiliation of the majority party in Congress. The cost of living and the cost of housing have increased dramatically. Of even greater concern is the relentless increase in the cost of quality medical care and the fact that our utilization of healthcare services over time will unquestionably increase as we move into and through retirement. Many of us will require some form of long-term care before we die. That can be extremely expensive.

In developing your retirement income plan, assume that you will require 100% of your maximum pre-retirement income. Be sure to consider the rapidly escalating cost of healthcare. If it turns out that the 100% assumption leaves you with excess monthly income, so be it. Donate the excess to the charity of your choice. You don't want to be cash-poor in retirement or outlive your resources entirely.

Find a way to stay involved in medicine or in some aspect of healthcare. At retirement, most physicians have been dedicated to clinical patient care and/or administration for more than three decades. It has been an all-consuming endeavor for most of us, enjoyable or not. We care deeply about our patients, our practices and employees, and the future path of the healthcare enterprise.

To assume that in retirement we will be happy to have no involvement whatsoever in healthcare may be an erroneous assumption. Most physicians are happier in retirement when they can maintain some connection to their previous working environment or carve out some new relationship to the world of healthcare in which they can leverage their many years of knowledge, experience, and ideas to improve systems of care.

By continuing to be involved in healthcare in some way, you will not only preserve a sense of contribution and meaning in your life, you will also stay connected to people who share your values and history. And, you will be helping people, the fundamental reason most of you chose a career in healthcare in the first place.

Find ways to keep your mind active and continuously learning. Physicians have spent their entire careers devoted to staying current in their field of practice. It is a practical necessity. Those who do not continually learn get weeded out of practice in a variety of ways. Keep your mind active, stimulated, and working to solve problems in retirement as well. Learning maintains the neural plasticity of your brain, elevates mood, delays cognitive decline with increasing age, and works to improve the health and functioning of the rest of your body.

ЁЁЁЁЁЁЁЁ

Develop and sustain physical fitness. The paradox of medicine is that doctors are dedicated to taking care of everyone except themselves. As a part of the culture of medical training, we finish training and enter the workplace with the belief—conscious or not—that our personal needs and feelings must always come second to those of our patients and colleagues.

Poor self-care is the primary explanation for the epidemic of professional burnout plaguing our profession in the United States and elsewhere in the developed world. We never learn how to take state-of-the-art care of ourselves. Attempts to do so typically lead to feelings of guilt or an inner belief that we are being self-centered. In reality, taking good care of ourselves is not self-centered, but self-centering.

Whether or not we have maintained good physical and emotional health during our working career, in retirement we have no excuses for not doing so. Regular aerobic exercise releases an endorphin response to sustain a positive mood and outlook on life. It also keeps our metabolism primed and our immune system working efficiently.

In retirement, we have the time to prioritize eight or more hours of sleep nightly. Stretching exercises, yoga, and weight training can help us reach and sustain a healthy lean body weight and maintain mobility and flexibility. We no longer have the excuse of being too busy and stressed to eat healthy.

In retirement, we minimize fast foods, unsaturated fats, and alcohol intake, and eat sugar and white flour products sparingly. To the extent we practice such a program of self-care, we are healthy, happy, and resilient to stress and disease.

Chapter 7 offers a discussion of strategies for work-life balance provides a more detailed prescription for maintaining physical, emotional, and spiritual health.

WHY SHOULD YOU RETIRE?

Here are some reasons you should consider retirement.

1. Because you can afford to retire.

This is the basic requirement for most physicians to consider retiring under non-emergent conditions. Defining how much in your retirement portfolio makes retirement "affordable" is defined earlier in this chapter.

2. You're satisfied with your career contributions.

For most physicians, the primary driver for choosing a career in medicine is to help people. For others, it's to contribute to society, to advance the forefront of science, or to have a stable dependable career that pays well. Some physicians never tire of their work even into their 70s and beyond.

At some point, however, many physicians reach a point at which they conclude that their original primary career goals have been fulfilled. They have done everything professionally that they wanted to accomplish. Rather than soldier on, they decide to enter a new stage in their lives and careers by retiring or moving on to a new business interest or new career.

3. You are confronting your/a love one's physical or mental health limitations.

Discussed in detail in Chapter 12, physical health may deteriorate, physical or mental disability or impairment may prevent a physician from performing optimally. These circumstances may create the necessity of retirement or career transition. These same problems can befall the spouse or partner of a physician, leading to a decision to leave practice in order to provide care to a loved one.

4. You have lost interest in the work.

See page 170 for a more detailed discussion of this topic.

5. You're chronically over-stressed despite serious attempts to overcome it.

Stress and burnout have become endemic in American physicians. Chapter 7 provides a detailed discussion of how best to prevent burnout and how work-life balance can heal professional burnout. Some physicians are resistant to treatment, as discussed on page 167. Those resistant to treatment, despite extensive effort and professional help, are candidates to leave practice and retire or transition to a new career.

6. You've been outpaced by technology.

In the past four decades, not only have advances in clinical care exploded, but so, too, has the technology that drives much of these advances. In no field is this truer than in diagnostic imaging. Since we completed training, the following have been developed and implemented into daily clinical practice:

- Real-time ultrasound
- Obstetrical ultrasound
- Magnetic resonance body imaging
- MR-angiography and cardiac imaging
- PET imaging
- PET-CT imaging
- Molecular imaging
- Cross-sectional image-guided interventions

- PACS systems of image storage and display
- Voice-activated dictation and reporting systems

Advances in these modalities come on a daily basis, and it's difficult if not impossible for a practicing clinical radiologist to stay abreast of all of these advances in imaging. It is even more difficult for clinicians who use imaging regularly to keep up. As a result, many physicians not practicing in large academic centers find themselves technologically behind. Once you get significantly behind, it becomes nearly impossible to catch up—and that may signal that it's time to retire.

7. You are unhappy with healthcare trends.

Physicians long ago gave up the helm of the healthcare ship. That's just a statement of fact. Management of healthcare by businesspeople, attorneys, and hospital administrators has led to many adverse developments for physicians and patients too extensive to attempt to catalogue here. You're familiar with all of them anyway.

8. You have a burning passion to start a new career or business.

Many physicians are entrepreneurs and inventors. Many are exceedingly good businesspeople. At some point in your career, you may develop a knockout idea for a new product or business that may or may not be connected to healthcare. The demands of a busy medical practice often put the kibosh on such ideas.

Some physicians are so taken by their idea, so passionate about bringing it to fruition, that they transition themselves to part-time clinical practice or, if finances permit, retire from practice to pursue their entrepreneurial project or to launch their new business. Although sometimes riskier than clinical practice, new business ventures and adventures can bring a fresh, positive and exciting perspective on life and career. The "juice of life" comes from taking risks occasionally.

WHICH PHYSICIANS *SHOULD* RETIRE?

Which physicians should retire even if they don't think they are ready?

1. Physicians with age-related cognitive impairment.

All of us experience some loss of cognitive function as we age—some of us more so than others. It is often the observations or comments of others that draw our attention to our declining clinical production, our declining ability to focus on the topic of the moment, our increasing difficulty remembering names, the proper doses of medication, or the name of the journal article we read last week. Gradually we become more aware of forgotten appointments, the names of friends and associates, and other things that in the past were instantly brought to mind.

These are all signals that our brain is no longer working at maximum efficiency and they should signal to a physician that it is time to hang up the spurs. Waiting too long puts your patients at risk of a medical error, can adversely affect their safety, and may increase your risk of malpractice litigation.

There are no easy laboratory tests or brain scans that will reliably tell you when it is time to stop practicing. When any signs of cognitive impairment become evident on a recurring basis, you should seriously consider retirement from clinical practice.

2. Physicians with chronic emotional and/or psychiatric disability.

Thanks to remarkable advances in psychopharmacology and psychotherapy over the past four decades, many debilitating emotional disorders can be reasonably well managed, keeping professionals working effectively. However, when psychosis is present, unresponsive to appropriate medical therapy, the ability of a doctor to practice medicine safely is compromised. Physicians with recurrent major depression not responsive to medical management are also compromised.

3. Physicians whose physical problems impair patient care.

Practicing at the peak of our game means we are consistently available for our patients, skilled at the procedures we perform, proactively updating our medical knowledge, and able to focus for long periods on our work and responsibilities.

Chronic medical or surgical problems may significantly affect physicians' performance of any or all of the above aspects of their work. Medications required to control disease or relieve pain may adversely affect our energy or clarity of thought. Having to be absent from our practice in order to see physicians taking care of us may negatively affect our ability to be available for our own patients and colleagues. These same issues may make taking night and emergency call difficult to impossible. When these situations persist, a physician should consider retiring from clinical practice.

4. Physicians with multiple adverse medical malpractice judgments.

Practicing medicine in the current milieu of escalating malpractice litigation requires courage, skill, and good luck. We are all at risk of making an error of commission or omission with every patient with whom we engage.

Over the course of their medical careers, approximately 50% of all American physicians are sued at least once for malpractice. The vast majority of these lawsuits are eventually dropped or are settled in favor of the physician, yet once a physician has been sued for malpractice, his or her risk of subsequent lawsuits increases significantly. The impacts of malpractice allegations are so devastating that a lawsuit almost always interferes with a physician's equanimity, self-confidence, and self-esteem. Those factors alone make a physician undergoing litigation more prone to making an error—which leads to an adverse patient event with the potential to become a second lawsuit. A detailed discussion of the implications and outcomes of malpractice is provided in Chapter 12.

There is a separate category of physicians who experience multiple lawsuits that may come in rapid succession. This situation should raise a red flag not only to physician practice groups, medical executive committees, and licensing agencies, but also to the physician himself/herself. Underlying this pattern of lawsuits may be unrecognized substance abuse or addiction, mental illness, and/or substandard medical knowledge, patient management skills, or technical skills.

If you have been involved in multiple malpractice suits, seek professional help to evaluate your mind and performance. If you don't have the capacity to be honest with yourself, then get out of clinical medicine for the sake of patient safety.

5. Physicians with untreatable addictions.

Physicians with chronic relapses and inability to maintain sobriety despite repeated in-patient treatment admissions and rigorous 12-Step recovery work should leave clinical practice. In fact, the State Medical Board and/or the State Physician Health Program often make that decision for the physician.

6. Physicians with chronic, unresponsive professional burnout.

Career burnout is not necessarily a fatal condition for a doctor's career—physicians can recover from it. That said, a small subset of burned-out physicians never succeed at recovery. They are unable or unwilling to do whatever needs to be done to recover. Physicians who have chronic, recurrent burnout that is resistant to treatment should give serious thought to retiring or transitioning to some new clinical or non-clinical field.

7. Physicians who have a compelling new life or career vision.

We all have fantasies of doing something else. Some physicians are inventors by nature and have ideas of how to make a better catheter, or a better surgical instrument, or something else. Some physicians want to turn their hobby into a new career. Others just want to exit from patient care but would like to remain involved in healthcare as a medical-legal consultant, administrator, or educator. We know physicians who have left clinical medicine to become chefs, radio/TV commentators, and poets.

If you find yourself reading literature about a career entirely different than your medical career, and in fact prefer to read those books over the medical literature in your field, pay attention! You would likely be much happier doing what you are passionately interested in rather than be bored or frustrated with your patient-care career.

Invest some time and money exploring those possibilities. Hire a career coach who specializes in working with physicians. See whether you have the appropriate skills, career values, and personality to succeed at your fantasy career. Do some informational interviews with people in the field you are considering.

Life is too short to spend it doing something you no longer want to do.

WHEN IS A GOOD TIME TO RETIRE?

When to retire is the million-dollar question. There probably are as many opinions about this topic as there are physicians thinking about retirement. Below are a few criteria for retirement that we believe are both practical and realistic.

1. You will know when it's time.

The simple truth is that when the right time comes, you will know it. It is an intuitive sense that you have come to the end of the road.

You wake up in the morning and the first thing that comes to your mind is how much you are dreading going into the office or hospital one more time. You have lost your sense of excitement about your work. You have lost the ability to be empathic with your patients.

"These are simply signs of professional burnout," you say. Yes, but somehow it will seem different this time. In your gut, you know it is time to leave medicine, and you are a bit surprised that you remain calm with this thought. No sense of fear, no regret. There is no one or nothing to blame. It is simply time.

2. Your retirement portfolio has sufficient value.

Not all physicians and certainly not all certified financial planners would agree on how much monetary value you need in your diversified retirement portfolio in order to feel comfortable retiring.

Here is a simple definition: You have enough when after thorough planning with your retirement planner, you have determined the cost in today's dollars of the lifestyle you want in retirement; you have made a very conservative estimate of the rate of return you expect on your portfolio for the duration of your retirement and the rate of inflation over the years of your retirement; you have confirmed that you can live the lifestyle you expect on an annual withdrawal of no more than 4% of your portfolio; and you have confirmed that using those criteria your money will last until you and/or your spouse/partner are least 90 years old.

3. At least one of the "why to retire" issues is present.

We previously listed several factors that constitute the "whys" to leave practice. When any of those factors is present in your life, a decision to retire from clinical practice can be justified, assuming that adequate financial assets are available. That does not mean that a retiring physician has no intention of working in some income-producing capacity after retiring from patient-care medicine.

4. Your professional life is no longer fun.

Chapter 1 addresses the four stages of the Career Cycle. In the first phase, Go For It, physicians are excited and stimulated with their work. It is so much fun you would nearly consider doing it for free. At the other end of a physician's career, that sense of excitement and stimulation may fade and eventually disappear. Although this happens slowly, awareness of it may come upon you suddenly. One morning you wake up when the alarm goes off and your first thought is, "I hate my job" or, "I have lost interest in my work."

Thoughts such as this can arise at any time of a physician's career. Thoughts and feelings of frustration, anger, wanting to quit, and helplessness to make things better may all be signs of professional burnout. When that is the case, working to combat your burnout typically reverses these sentiments and feelings to a large degree or completely.

After devoting serious time and effort to dealing with these symptoms of burnout, including working with a physician career professional, if your work is pervasively a drudge, not fun, and a consistent source of negative emotions and stress, it is time to give serious thought to retirement or leaving this kind of work for something else of greater interest and meaning.

5. You are still healthy.

Our most important asset is our health. Without it, nothing goes the way we prefer. When we are young, we tend to take our good health for granted—we think ourselves invulnerable to the serious diseases and injuries that we treat every day as physicians. Of course, doctors are equally as susceptible to sickness, disease, mental illness, and trauma as the general population.

We all know the story of the professional athlete who has difficulty leaving his fame and his sport behind only to be forced to retire by a serious injury. The same thing regularly happens to physicians: premature retirement brought on by unexpected disease, injury, or disability.

When possible, physicians should retire while they are still healthy and vigorous. That doesn't mean they have to leave patient care completely. Maybe they work less than full-time. Maybe they volunteer their time in a clinic for the medically underserved. The point is after working so hard for so long, it is sad to see some physicians become disabled, develop a debilitating illness, or die from a massive coronary only six months prior to their planned retirement.

Retire in time to enjoy the fruits of your labor! Be good to yourself—you deserve it.

PROTIREMENT PLANNING: BEWARE OF UNEXPECTED PITFALLS

Beware of these unexpected obstacles to a happy protirement.

1. Loss of self-identity, confusion, anxiety, and depression.

After decades of clinical practice, physicians are accustomed to regular positive feedback assuring us that we are smart, empathic, caring, kind, creative, and funny. That kind of positive support and affirmation often stops when the physician stops going to the office, clinic, or hospital. Suddenly there are no patients to tell us how wonderful we are. There are no curbside consults with colleagues in need of our special expertise. The employees who valued our guidance and mentoring are no longer a part of our daily routine.

It should be no surprise that the sudden withdrawal of these forms of ego satisfaction and support lead to negative consequences for many retired physicians relative to their mood, self-esteem, and outlook. In our experience, these unanticipated consequences of retirement may become apparent within weeks and certainly within months of retirement from practice for some of us.

What to do? As part of protirement planning, it is important for physicians to incorporate activities into their retirement life plan that will bring them into regular daily contact with friends, other retired physicians, family members and other loved ones, and people we may interact with through our volunteering to help others. These daily human interactions are crucial for our happiness, sense of well-being, and self-esteem. The positive feedback previously associated primarily with patients and colleagues will be replaced by the positive interactions with a new set of people and circumstances. Those who are successful at this transition are happier and tend not to become confused, depressed, or lonely.

2. Boredom.

The practice of medicine is endlessly challenging, stimulating, and demanding of all of our personal resources. In retirement, we must look elsewhere for sources of healthy physical and emotional challenges, excitement, and intellectual stimulation. While many of us happily anticipate playing golf or tennis with friends multiple times a week to keep us busy, our experience is that physicians quickly get bored doing just that. As you prepare for retirement, consider and plan for specific activities and people with which to engage your body, mind, and spirit.

3. Loneliness.

During our practice years, our days are filled with work from dawn until dusk, and often late into the night. There is often little time for us to eat, chat with a friend, or daydream. That said, we are constantly interacting with patients, partners at work, support staff, and administrators. While not all of those daily interactions are fun or relaxing, they do keep us engaged in our world of patient care.

Retired physicians no longer have those daily interactions with other healthcare professionals or patients. They devoted so much time and energy to their practices that most have few if any intimate friends. Thus, once retired, they have a very small social network and may become lonely.

The solution, again, is to begin planning long before actual retirement how and with whom to interact, with whom to develop new friendships, and with whom to pursue fun.

4. Lack of meaning and ego satisfaction.

Whether you were consciously aware of it or not, your medical career provided a great deal of meaning to your life. Helping others, after all, is the most common motivation for becoming physicians, according to medical students. Once you step away from clinical medicine, the major source of meaning in your life disappears and so do the many sources of ego satisfaction and human interaction.

One of the keys to maintaining happiness in retirement is finding suitable ways to replace those lost sources of meaning and ego satisfaction. During your protirement planning phase, consider activities and relationships that you would enjoy, that would be meaningful to you, and that would provide ample opportunities for interpersonal interaction.

Many physicians find such opportunities in the realm of volunteering, public service, teaching, shared hobbies, consulting, social activities with other retired friends, and active lifestyles outside of the home environment. This topic is discussed in greater detail in Chapter 7.

5. Friction at home.

Your retirement is something you and your spouse or partner likely have been looking forward to for a long time. However, once retirement day arrives, things at home undergo an important change. For one thing, you are at home a great deal more than usual. As the old saying goes, "you marry for better or worse, but not for lunch."

You engage your partner in conversation, suggest activities you can do together every day, take control of the remote. Rather than basking in the new blissful home life, your spouse or partner becomes irritable or inattentive, or devises errands to take him or her out of the house—without you.

What happened? You intruded on your partner's routine, private time, alone time. You've disrupted what was likely a very comfortable daily routine.

This is the challenge of married/partnership relationships in retirement. Use your protirement planning time to anticipate and address this question together long before your retirement date. Talk about how much time you wish to spend together and how you are going to do that. Discuss how much alone time you each need and how you will manage that. Clarify how you will communicate your needs to be alone or together. In so doing, you will be showing respect for each other, enhancing your intimacy, and avoid having to guess what your spouse is thinking.

ADDITIONAL FINANCIAL CONSIDERATIONS

Retiring physicians often face unexpected expenses or find that their financial situation won't provide for the comfortable life they expected. This was all too common for many physicians with investments that all but disappeared during the economic downturn that began in 2008.

Physicians contemplating retirement within a few years need to understand the future risks of the financial situation they may be facing. People are living longer, which means you may have to provide for a bigger cushion in retirement than you may have initially intended. In addition, uncertainty over future Social Security benefits as Baby Boomers continue to retire adds to the concerns. As a result, you could face a personal shortfall, especially if you incur unforeseen expenses from a medical condition or some other unanticipated situation.

What could/should you do? Even if retirement is imminent, you may be able to make up lost ground quickly or take other steps to protect yourself. Here are several ideas to consider:

- **Maximize retirement savings vehicles.** Just a few years of making contributions at or near the maximum level can significantly bolster your account. If you have any qualified retirement plans that you are not fully funding, determine if your cash flow will allow you to do so.

- **Work on the budget.** If a financial planning retirement needs analysis determines that you may have a potential shortfall, you might want to dial down your expectations. Make realistic estimates about the income you expect to have coming in and the expenses going out. Although you will likely be paying less for housing (see below) and other items such as life insurance, especially if your children are already adults, consider the impact of potential increases in some expenses such as travel expenditures and healthcare.

- **Move to a smaller home or condo.** For most people, housing is the largest overall cost, representing on average more than one-third of overall spending. If your kids no longer live with you, but you're still living in the large home where you raised them, it may be time to downsize. In addition, you might want to move to a state with a different climate, taking state income taxes into account. Various other factors such as proximity to family and personal preferences may also come into play.

- **Refinance your current home.** If you decide not to downsize, you should consider refinancing an existing mortgage if you are paying a rate higher than those currently available. At the beginning of 2013, mortgage rates had reached historic lows. Even though rates have increased slightly since then, you may save tens of thousands of dollars over time by refinancing. Keep in mind that your interest payments will generally continue to be tax-deductible.

- **Do not stop working altogether: Just because you have reached retirement age does not mean you have to stop working completely.** If needed, you could pursue part-time employment. For some individuals, working full-time a little longer is also a viable option. For a more detailed discussion of options to work for income in retirement refer to Chapter 13.

THE FINAL STEPS IN CLOSING YOUR PRACTICE

1. Notify your state medical society of your intent to retire and the official date.
2. Notify your patients of your plan to retire and specific date. You should give them ample time to find another physician. Provide patients an opportunity to have their records transferred to another physician. You may wish to recommend a list of potential physicians to whose care they may wish to transfer.
3. Notify your office staff of your plan to retire and the date. Your employees will need to find new employment after you retire, and you obviously want to give them ample time to seek and find new employment.
4. Arrange for storage of your medical records and practice business records. Most states require you to retain all patient medical records for a minimum of seven years. If another doctor takes over your practice, he or she must agree to keep those records on your behalf. With the use of electronic medical

records, this requirement will be much easier than paying for storage of paper files.

5. Notify your malpractice insurance carrier of your retirement date. We recommend purchasing tail coverage (as opposed to occurrence-based coverage) to ensure that you and your practice will be covered in the event a malpractice claim is filed against you after you have retired.

6. Check your office lease and be certain that you have the right to sublet. Then obtain a release from further liability for rent and damages from your landlord.

7. Plan the sale of your practice. If you are in a partnership with other physicians, you may have a buy/sell agreement in place that provides for the buyout of a retiring partner. If you are in solo practice, you may wish to hire a broker to sell your practice or take in an associate for a year or two prior to retirement with the intent that the associate will buy the practice upon your retirement. The sale of your practice was discussed in greater detail in Chapter 13.

8. Be sure that final statements from suppliers and vendors have been paid.

9. Change your office mailing address at your local post office and cancel journal subscriptions you no longer want to receive.

SUMMARY

Retirement from the practice of medicine requires many skills and a long timeline. Ideally the planning should begin in the early phase of a physician's career. It is better to "protire" than retire. By that we mean that a physician should begin proactively planning what you would like your life to look like after practice, how and where you would like to live, how you want to spend your time, what that lifestyle will cost in dollars based on assumptions about inflation, and then working with a certified financial planner to develop a well thought out retirement plan and an income plan to support the life and lifestyle you envision.

We have provided guidelines for why to retire, who should retire, when to retire, and some of the pitfalls which you may encounter along the way. Finally, some practical tasks to complete in closing your practice to patients.

Following the guidelines for "protirement" will serve you well, and provide you with a satisfying sense of solid preparation as the day for you to leave clinical practice draws near.

CHAPTER 14

Selling Your Practice

Randy Bauman*

PHYSICIANS IN THE LATER STAGES of their careers who have maintained their independence and resisted selling their practice often have a renewed interest in selling as they near retirement. This interest may be motivated by a desire to realize some value for their practice but it also is often driven by the desire to assure some level of continuity of care for their patients as well.

Selling can be a good option and in many cases may be the only option. Recruiting a younger physician to buy into and take over your practice may have been an option in earlier generations, but the current generation of younger physicians has less interest in the business side of medicine and tends to be more averse to financial risks. Often the options come down to either selling or closing the practice.

THE UNIVERSE OF POTENTIAL PURCHASERS

The universe of potential purchasers generally consists of existing associates or partners, younger physicians seeking to start or build a practice, existing single and multispecialty group practices, and hospitals/health systems. Let's take a closer look at each.

Existing Associates or Partners

If you are fortunate enough to have a newly recruited associate or existing partner, the buy-out terms typically were established on the front end, when that physician formally signed on or became a partner. Problem solved, right? Unfortunately no, this situation can present issues, too.

Upon your retirement, the remaining physician or physicians may face several economic issues that can affect you as well.

If the remaining physician or physicians have full practices, when you retire, regardless of the buy-out terms, they will lack the capacity to continue to serve all your patients. Recruiting a replacement for you needs to be planned well in

---

*Author's Note: some of the content of this chapter was excerpted from my book, *Time To Sell—Guide to Selling a Physician Practice*, third edition, Greenbranch Publishing 2016.

advance because recruiting is difficult in many parts of the country and many young physicians prefer straight employment over becoming an associate on a partnership track. They have extensive debt and want to be certain of a regular paycheck and avoid uncertainty and penalties associated with paying down their medical school and training loans.

While you already have existing agreements regarding retirement and the sale of your ownership interest in the practice upon retirement, in many cases, these agreements were written years ago and may not accurately reflect the ability and intention of the remaining physicians. Two issues often arise in this situation: payment of the buyout and increased practice overhead.

Buyout payments usually involve the value for the furniture and equipment and the value of the accounts receivable. Sometimes buyouts include additional payments for intangible or goodwill value as well. The payment of these obligations, depending on how the payments are structured, can present a severe financial stress on the remaining physicians and may exceed what the remaining physicians can or are willing to absorb.

Increased practice overhead results because most overhead costs in a medical practice are fixed. Rent, for example, doesn't go down when one physician retires unless the remaining physicians are able to move into smaller space or renegotiate the lease, which is often difficult or impossible. Staffing, sans perhaps a medical assistant or nurse, probably won't decrease much either.

These two factors leave the remaining physicians with increased per-physician overhead layered with the payment of buyout obligations.

In the past, these factors could be overcome by recruiting a replacement physician, but in the current environment, the starting salary expectations and willingness and ability of the younger physicians to assume financial risk will likely make recruiting difficult if not impossible.

Ultimately, the financial resources of the group may not mesh with the existing agreements and many times these issues lead the practice to seek assistance from a local hospital. This assistance typically comes in two forms: an outright sale or recruiting support coupled with an income guarantee to a newly recruited physician.

Many hospitals will offer recruiting support and income guarantees to private practices as an alternative to purchasing the practice. Typically, under an income guarantee arrangement, the hospital will provide and pay for recruiting a new physician and guarantee the income of that physician for a period of one to two years. The income guarantee usually covers a predetermined monthly collection amount plus the incremental overhead the practice incurs as a result of the new physician—actually writing a check to the practice monthly to cover any shortfalls.

The income guarantee usually is structured as a loan that is forgiven over a period of years, typically two to three years, after the guarantee expires.

All of this may sound attractive, but it does present some issues that are often troublesome to younger physicians. Legally, the loan obligation is an obligation of the young physician, basically requiring him or her to stay in the practice until the loan is forgiven. Many young physicians prefer to avoid a commitment of four or five years and that commitment is often coupled with becoming a partner in the group after the guarantee period (typically two years) is over. As noted above, since younger physicians are mostly eschewing private practice for hospital employment, an income guarantee that puts them in a private practice may simply not be sellable.

On the positive side, assuming the right candidate can be found, the practice can maintain its independence while reaping the benefits the hospital guarantee provides. Hospitals have a better chance of recruiting a physician because they have deeper pockets—they can afford to pay the recruiting fees and offer market salaries, signing bonuses, student loan repayment, moving expense reimbursement, and other benefits that independent groups find difficult to afford without the income guarantee.

Younger Physicians Seeking to Start or Build a Practice

Younger physicians starting and building a private practice are generally in short supply. Many are laden with medical school debt and in recent years have been more interested in working for hospitals and health systems. They tend to be uninterested in the business side of medicine and are risk-averse.

A few years ago, I worked with a well-respected primary care physician who was in his mid-60s and contemplating retirement. He was negotiating with a young physician down the street who was just getting started about selling his practice and wasn't making much progress so he brought my company in to try to move things along.

"He's 64 years old," the younger physician told me, "why should I pay him for his practice when I can run a newspaper ad in about six months and pick up most of it for free?"

This response illustrates a key point: the closer you get to retirement, the less value your practice will have. The younger physician wasn't wrong. The reality is that when you retire, your patients will find another physician one way or another.

So plan ahead, start shopping early, and try to keep your plans close to the vest if you want to try to maintain your value.

Absent a viable succession plan in your private practice—existing partners or newly recruited associates interested in buying in to the practice and buying you out—selling to a hospital may be your only real viable option.

Existing Single and Multispecialty Groups

Existing single or multispecialty groups are other options for selling your practice. While these groups don't exist in every community, those that do have often grown through merger or acquisition with established practices.

These groups usually have some of the same advantages as hospitals. They often have the financial resources, size, and stability to attract and recruit young physicians. While younger physicians may eschew small private practices, there is a level of attraction that comes with joining a large single or multispecialty group: working with like-minded peers and colleagues in an independent setting that has the financial resources necessary to compete in the marketplace with larger hospitals and health systems.

The bad news is that such groups generally attract other physicians through increased income rather than through payment of large purchase prices. As you look toward retirement, increased income is likely not your main focus—you want to realize some value for your practice.

Most larger group practices have a great deal of flexibility in their acquisition model and can move much more quickly than a hospital. Where synergies can be demonstrated and a transaction benefits both parties, in the right situation they can be a viable option worth considering.

Hospitals and Health Systems

All things considered, hospitals generally represent the best option in the universe of potential purchasers for a retiring physician. While you may not want to be employed by a hospital, in order to maximize the value from your practice, it may be necessary and even a good way to wind down your career.

This is where timing can have an impact on your value. Rather than just announcing your pending retirement, develop an outline of a transition plan and present it to potential hospital suitors two or three years in advance. A successful transition plan needs to allow plenty of time for execution.

A typical transition plan involves the following:

1. Sale of your practice to the hospital.

2. Joint recruitment by you and the hospital of a physician. You and the hospital work together to jointly recruit a physician to replace you upon retirement. This step can be in process or even take place before the sale.
3. You continue in practice as a hospital employee while the new physician is recruited and for a period of time afterward during which you gradually reduce your work level and consciously and deliberately transition your patients to the new physician.

If you are fortunate enough to practice in a community where there are two or more hospitals in heated competition, it may be possible to push the envelope on the sales price by creating competition for your practice. However, as discussed below, hospitals are highly regulated with respect to what they can pay for a practice.

THE CYLE OF PHYSICIAN EMPLOYMENT

Another thing to be aware of when considering selling to a hospital is that the employment of physicians by hospitals tends to be cyclical. Physicians seeking to sell their practices and become hospital employees should be consciously aware that the hospital acquisition and employment of physicians seems to be repeating the same cycle we saw in the 1990s. In its basic form, the cycle has three phases: Phase 1: Acquisition, Phase 2: Operational Development, and Phase 3: Restructuring/Divestiture. This cycle is illustrated in Figure 14-1.

Assessing where the local healthcare market or hospital is within this cycle can provide valuable insight to physicians who are considering the sale of their practice.

Phase 1 usually represents the best time to sell your practice. It is characterized by rapid acquisition, often with little time to give thought to development of the proper infrastructure to operate the employed practices. Physicians who are considering selling their practice to a hospital that is in this phase are in the "sweet spot."

Contract terms and compensation are more negotiable; the drive is often to do whatever needs to be done to "get the deal done." In competitive markets, prices hospitals offer often include intangible assets and even goodwill, whereas

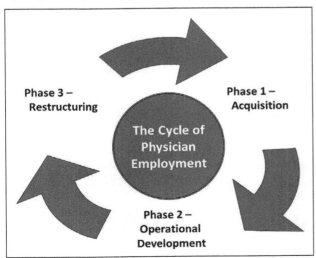

Figure 14-1. The Cycle of Physician Employment.

hospitals in noncompetitive markets will generally eschew these items and only offer to acquire furniture, fixtures, and equipment.

For physicians who are planning to practice a few more years before retirement, compensation plans and models typically aren't standardized at this phase. Compensation offers tend to be more aggressive and compensation tends to be higher. Compensation models are less structured and often vary widely, even between physicians in the same specialty employed by the same hospital.

Phase 2 is generally characterized by evolving the operation of standalone physician offices to a more consolidated and standardized group practice platform. Hospitals expect to lose money employing physicians, and as Phase 2 of the cycle unfolds, they usually find the losses to be much higher than anticipated.

While hospitals continue to acquire practices at this stage, acquisition prices and compensation structures become more standardized and less aggressive as they struggle to realize cost efficiencies and reduce losses. In the later stages of Phase 2, hospitals begin to experience "leakage." "Leakage," refers to the departure of physicians who, for whatever reason (usually economic) decide that hospital employment doesn't work for them.

Phase 3 often usually begins as an often-frenetic attempt by the hospital to reduce operating losses and restructure the employed physician network. Hospitals rarely enter Phase 3 with the focus of divestiture, but that is sometimes the outcome. Often this phase results in deliberate divestiture of underperforming practices or reductions in physician compensation that leave physicians looking for other options.

Hospitals in Phase 3 often have tepid interest in additional acquisitions but will do so in the right circumstance.

Keeping your ear to the ground, talking to your peers and colleagues, and generally being aware of what is going on within your local market hospitals with respect to employing physicians can help you determine where they are in this cycle. This can give you some insight into how they might approach the purchase of your practice and allow you to gauge their interest.

Currently most hospitals are in the late stages of Phase 2, but we've seen some hospitals in the early stages of Phase 1 and some are well into Phase 3.

PRACTICE VALUATION—WHAT IS YOUR PRACTICE WORTH?

If you decide to try to sell to an existing single or multispecialty group, understand that they are not subject to the same regulations as hospitals and, as noted above, likely have their own valuation and acquisition models that can be flexible to your situation.

If you decide to further explore the sale of your practice to a hospital, the process is likely to be more formal. Typically, the hospital will engage an independent firm—chosen and paid for by the hospital—to assess your practice and arrive at a fair market value.

You will be asked to share extensive financial and operating data. Providing complete and accurate data is important. Incomplete documentation tends to reduce the value of a practice because absent documentation, the valuation firm is likely to make the most conservative assumptions.

Valuation Components

The value of any business, including physician practices, generally consists of two types of assets: tangible and intangible.

Tangible assets in a physician practice consist of furniture and equipment, inventory and supplies, and accounts receivable (A/R). Many practices also own the practice's facility, often through a separate real estate entity that leases the facility to the practice.

Intangible assets include things like an established patient base, reputation of the physician(s), an established referral base, a trained workforce, patient medical records, and the name and phone number of the practice. Intangible assets are often referred to as "goodwill."

A valuation worksheet is provided at the end of this chapter to assist you in estimating the value of your practice for comparison to the hospital's valuation.

Valuation of Tangible Assets

Furniture and Equipment

Furniture and equipment will be valued at less than your original cost but probably more than their current net book value for tax purposes, which is simply the original cost less the total depreciation you have been allowed to deduct on your tax return since you purchased the asset.

Tax law generally allows depreciating assets over a fairly short period of time—generally a much shorter time than the actual period the asset will be used in the practice; therefore, net book value is generally going to understate the actual value of your furniture and equipment.

The appraisers will ask for or take a physical inventory that lists all the furniture and equipment in your practice, including description, make and model, date acquired, and original cost of the major items. Sometimes this information can be obtained from a depreciation schedule—a work paper your CPA firm maintains for use in preparing your tax return. Depreciation schedules are often incomplete and out of date, so make sure you review yours and update it as needed. If the appraiser asks you to complete a physical inventory, take the time to provide complete and accurate information.

The value of furniture and equipment is generally determined through secondary market prices or as a percent of what is called standard replacement cost.

The value of items that are of a more specialized nature such as exam tables, and expensive medical equipment (such as x-ray and ultrasound machines or lab and other diagnostic or treatment equipment) is often determined based on the secondary or used equipment market. The Internet provides easy access to dozens of used equipment vendors as well as other marketplaces such as eBay. These items are generally valued at the prices for which functionally similar equipment is for sale or recently sold in the secondary market.

Items of a more generic nature that are not readily available in the secondary market are often valued at a percent of standard replacement cost. Standard replacement cost is the appraiser's estimate of the replacement cost of furnishing a physician office with equipment of like utility. The value is generally a percent of the standard replacement cost based on the age and condition of your furniture and equipment.

A rule of thumb to estimate the value of a practice's furniture and equipment is to take net book value and add back 50% of the accumulated depreciation shown on your balance sheet. Your CPA can help you with this calculation if necessary, or you can try it yourself using the worksheet at the end of this chapter. While this method will not be totally accurate, it will give you a rough idea of the value to expect.

Make sure you exclude from your estimate, assets that tend to be more personal in nature. The hospital likely won't be interested in purchasing any antique furniture, original artwork, or practice-owned vehicles.

Accounts Receivable (A/R)

Accounts receivable represents work you've already done and, while a tangible asset of your practice, is usually not part of the transaction. If a hospital does purchase A/R, which is extremely rare, it will do so at a discounted rate and then attempt to collect (and keep) what it gets post-sale. In most instances, it's better for both parties if the physician keeps the outstanding A/R. Hospitals will usually allow your billing staff, who become their employees after the sale, to spend some time each week for a few months collecting your A/R.

A rule of thumb for estimating the value of A/R is to take the total balance of A/R outstanding less than 60 days and multiply it by your practice's historical gross collection rate. In most practices, the value should be equal to between one and two months' worth of collections. Here again, this method will not be totally accurate, but it will give you a rough idea of the value to expect.

Inventory and Supplies

Inventory and supplies generally are not a significant component of the tangible value. If you have an extensive inventory of drugs and supplies, it will be to your benefit to provide copies of recent invoices to aid the hospital in assigning a fair value to these items.

The rule of thumb here is to estimate the value by adding your average annual costs for office and medical supplies and drugs and multiplying by .17. This equates to about two months' worth of annual expense in inventory, which again, should provide a reasonable estimate.

Real Estate

Many practices own their own office building, generally in an entity separate from the practice entity. This asset, while not technically part of your practice's value, often represents the majority of your investment and is a key consideration in your decision to sell.

Many hospitals simply will not purchase physician-owned real estate. Instead, they will offer to lease the office space at a fair market value rental rate. If this is the hospital's approach, be sure the lease term is long enough to adequately provide you with a rental income stream to cover any mortgage payments and that there is clear agreement on things like taxes, insurance, repairs, and maintenance.

Some hospitals will purchase real estate, especially if it is in a desirable location. Here, too, the hospital will engage an independent third-party appraiser (often a different appraiser than the one who valued the practice) and will be bound by the appraiser's valuation. If you don't feel the appraisal reflects the fair value of the facility or, as has often been the case in recent years, you feel the value is depressed as a result of the economy, leasing the facility to the hospital for a few years with a "put" option can provide the best of both worlds. A put option requires the hospital to purchase the office at some future date for its appraised value at that time.

Another option that many hospitals offer is to put you in touch with a third-party investor or real estate developer who might purchase your real estate.

Valuation of Intangible Assets

The value of tangible assets, with the exception of real estate, usually does not represent the bulk of what a physician thinks the practice is worth. Most physicians have the expectation of value in the intangible assets or what is commonly known as goodwill.

Physicians tend to think their practices are worth more than they actually are. Their first argument is usually how much revenue the practice generates for the hospital by admitting patients and making referrals for diagnostic testing and therapeutic care. This is an easy one to set aside: It is illegal for a hospital to factor this in, and no reputable hospital would do so.

The second argument is that there has to be value in the practice's goodwill. After all, returning patients; the reputation of the doctors, trained providers, and staff; an established referral base; medical records; and even the name and phone number of the practice are what make the practice a viable business, so those things have to have value.

While this goodwill does exist, the reality is that in the sale of a practice, it often has little or no value because that value is almost always paid out to the physician owners in salary and bonus annually, and this will generally continue after the sale.

The value of almost any business is in the future earnings stream that the business can be expected to generate for its owner. In this case, the owner will be the hospital. If the earnings stream the practice generates for the hospital is paid out to the physicians in salary and bonus, as the theory goes, there is no earnings stream on which to base the value.

Another way to think of this is that you are, in effect, benefiting from the goodwill of the practice each year through the earnings it generates for you.

This intangible value is even more at risk for a physician who is retiring. As discussed earlier in this chapter, any value in the patients will disappear rapidly as your imminent retirement becomes known because patients will seek care elsewhere.

While the prospect that your practice may have no goodwill value may be surprising and disappointing, if you step back and think about it, it makes sense. Why would anyone purchase a practice without a reasonable expectation of generating a profit from its investment? As noted above, the hospital cannot consider the value of any referrals because that would squarely be at odds with federal law.

Entire books have been written on valuing physician practices. Practice brokers and dozens of firms are on the Internet offering, for a price or commission, to tell you what your practice is worth and to help you sell it. If you are going to sell to a hospital, don't bother with these services. It doesn't matter what these firms tell you—the hospital is bound by the value determined by its independent appraiser and no more.

Another poor source of information on the value of your practice is the Internet. We recently were asked to value a practice owned by two nurse practitioners. The NPs told the hospital that, "according to their Internet research," their practice was worth $1 million. While it turned out to be a robust practice with good financial performance, it still had little or no goodwill value because they expected to continue (or even increase) their incomes after the sale, leaving no profit or return on investment for the purchaser.

Historically, many hospitals, both for-profit and not-for-profit, have taken an even more conservative approach: They simply have a policy against paying for intangible assets or goodwill—period. In many areas of the country, especially in the early stages of the current practice acquisition/sale trend, physicians were approaching hospitals, which indicated that in these areas it was a buyer's market. In a buyer's market, there is no compelling reason to pay for intangible assets or goodwill regardless of the practice's value. While this trend is still present in many markets, as further discussed below, in some markets this is changing.

Even in areas where there is competition among hospitals for practices, CEOs and hospital board members remember the lessons from the 1990s. Many simply are not willing to expose their hospital (or their job security) to repeating past mistakes.

Valuation Trends

Even the highly regulated healthcare marketplace is subject to market pressures driven by the law of supply and demand. As noted above, the early stages of the current trend of hospitals acquiring physician practices was driven primarily by physicians. In many markets, this led to a buyer's market and allowed hospitals to hide behind policies of "no goodwill."

As happened in the 1990s, when competition among hospitals heated up, prices for physician practices started to rise. While hospitals cannot pay more than fair market value determined by an independent third-party appraiser, in some areas market competition has led to a relaxation of these "no goodwill" policies.

We currently are seeing few hospitals pay for goodwill per se, but some are willing to pay for medical records and a trained workforce in place.

Hospital policies on payment for intangible assets vary widely, and some hospitals are changing those policies out of competitive necessity in markets where competition for physician practices is heating up and the market is shifting from a buyer's market to more of a seller's market.

This is where gaining a basic understanding of where your target hospital is in the cycle of physician employment described earlier in this chapter can give you some insight.

Holding On

The last thing to consider as you reach this stage of your career is whether you actually want to retire. I have worked with hundreds of physicians in my career and there is a sizable subset who are always "slowing down" or "getting ready to retire" but have a hard time actually taking that step.

There is nothing wrong with continuing to practice as long as your health, skills, and abilities permit it. As noted earlier, a majority of the overhead in a physician practice is fixed so that as volume and revenue drop as a physician cuts back and slows down to an increasingly part-time practice, the reduction comes right out of the bottom line. I looked at a practice recently where the physician had cut back by about 50% and his income had dropped to below $10,000 per year. At his age (he was 70) the income he earned wasn't all that important—he wanted something to do and wasn't ready to let go.

As I said, while there's nothing wrong with this approach, the value of his practice had diminished quite a bit because half of his patient base had already migrated to other physicians. In many situations such as this it is much more viable from a solely economic perspective to pursue such a "slow down" under the umbrella of an existing single or multi-specialty group or a hospital.

Practice Valuation Worksheets

These worksheets can provide a simple tool for estimating the value of your practice. These are estimates only and will likely vary from the hospital's valuation. They should be used to highlight differences between the actual value of your practice and your estimate, and as an aid in raising questions for discussion with the hospital.

TANGIBLE ASSETS

Furniture, Fixtures, and Equipment (FF&E)	Practice Estimate	Hospital Value
Cost		
– Accumulated depreciation		
= Net book value		
+ 50% of accumulated depreciation		
= Estimated Value of FF&E		

Accounts Receivable	Practice Estimate	Hospital Value
Accounts receivable outstanding less than 60 days		
– Practice's gross collection percentage (collections divided by gross charges for the past year)		
= Estimated Value of Accounts Receivable		

Inventory and Supplies	Practice Estimate	Hospital Value
Office supplies expense last year		
+ Medical supplies expense last year		
+ Vaccine and drug expense last year		
= Total drug and supply expense		
× Total by .1667 = Estimated Value		

Practice Value Summary	Practice Estimate	Hospital Value
Total Estimated Practice Value		
–Estimated Value of FF&E		
–Estimated Value of Accounts Receivable		
- Estimated Value of Inventory and Supplies		
= Intangible Value (if negative number, intangible (goodwill) value is zero)		

INTANGIBLE ASSETS

Note: Some hospitals will pay for the intangible assets listed below. Many will not under any circumstances.

Medical Records	Practice Estimate	Hospital Value
Number of Active Patient Charts (patients seen within the past 12 months)		
× $15.00 = Estimated Value		

Trained Workforce in Place	Practice Estimate	Hospital Value
Total Salary and Benefit Costs (exclude physician owners but include employed physicians and mid-level providers)		
× 20% = Estimated Value		

CHAPTER 15

Evolving Estate and Practice Priorities

Joel M. Blau and Ronald J. Paprocki

E VEN AS YOU LOOK BACK on your medical career, you need to look forward financially. Now is the time in your life to assess your financial situation and determine the impact the markets have had both positively and negatively on your long-term goals. Physicians who rely on guidance from professionals need to be certain that those relationships are based on mutual respect and on trust.

The relationship with one's financial advisor is a true partnership in which both parties are working toward a common goal: your financial stability and financial independence. Many retirees continue to work with their long-time advisors, while others look toward change. Change may be necessary to meet the challenges you will face in your retirement years. One of those changes may involve your choice of advisor as you move from active career business toward retirement. Is the advisor your own age, older, younger? If that advisor retires or dies, have you met the person who will become responsible for your financial planning?

Regardless whether you stay with your long-time advisor or find a new one, you should take the following steps to ensure you are receiving the full benefit of such a relationship and that you and your advisor are working together to meet your current and future financial goals.

- Evaluate your portfolio at least annually. Even if you work with an out-of-town advisor, it is important to put aside time on the phone or in person to review past performance and to discuss changes in goals or other life circumstances that may affect your future investing habits. Perhaps you have become more conservative and you want your portfolio to be realigned to better mirror your new risk tolerance. Any major changes could have tax implications. Before making any portfolio changes, your advisor should determine its tax ramifications.
- Be specific when communicating with your advisor about your financial goals and be open to constructive input. The best way to guarantee that your portfolio continues to support your objectives is to talk openly and frankly about

your objectives. Let your advisor know exactly what you expect concerning your investments and make sure you are comfortable with your choices.

- Read your mail. Don't discount investment materials as junk mail. Many of these materials provide valuable information that affects your portfolio. The more you read, the more you'll learn about your investments as well as other investment options. If you have questions about the materials, speak with your advisor.
- Ask your advisor questions. If you read or hear something you don't understand—ask. It's really your responsibility to let the advisor know what you need.
- Expect the market to continue to fluctuate. Advisors cannot eliminate market fluctuations, but they can design and implement strategies to minimize volatility.

As they approach retirement, many physicians wonder how much they will spend on various activities and living the lifestyle that they have envisioned for themselves. Spending levels typically are based on the three basic phases of the retirement years:

1. An active phase, when the retiree is in good health and actively pursues travel and hobbies. This is typically the most expensive phase.
2. A passive phase, when the retiree's energy starts to wane. Life starts to slow down and living expenses typically go down.
3. A final phase, when medical conditions often result in subsistence living. This is typically a more expensive time than the passive phase due to increased medical expenses, but as long as proper medical arrangements have been made in advance, this phase will probably not be as expensive as the active phase.

How much money do you need to retire? That's often the hottest topic discussed in physician lounges around the country. Many use online tools; others simply make a guess based on what colleagues or relatives have done or what they have read or seen in various financial media. However, no general guideline applies to every physician and every circumstance; each individual's situation is unique.

To enjoy your retirement without financial worries, you must ensure you have enough money saved based on your own unique circumstance. A variety of factors affect your analysis, and inaccurate estimates for any one of them can leave you with too little in savings.

RETIREMENT INCOME NEEDS

Various rules of thumb indicate you need retirement income ranging from 60% to more than 100% of your pre-retirement income. On the surface, it seems like you should need less than the higher amount because your expenses should be less in retirement if you have managed your finances appropriately during your years of gainfully practicing medicine.

Before deciding how much you'll need, look carefully at your current expenses and how you plan to spend your retirement. If you pay off your mortgage, stay in good health, live in a city with a low cost of living, and engage in inexpensive hobbies, then you might get by with less than 100% of your income. However, if you travel extensively and go first class and stay in 5-star hotels, pay for health insurance, and maintain significant debt levels, even 100% of your income may not be enough. Take a close look at your current expenses and planned retirement activities to come up with a reasonable estimate.

RETIREMENT AGE

When you retire determines how much time you have in which to save and how long investment returns can compound. Many physicians would like to retire before age 65, but that typically requires significant personal savings. You must be sure your retirement savings and other income sources, such as Social Security and pension benefits, will support you for what could be a lengthy retirement. Even postponing your retirement by a couple of years can significantly affect the ultimate amount you need.

LIFE EXPECTANCY

In predicting the length of their retirement, most people consider average life expectancy. Keep in mind that an average life expectancy means you have a 50% chance of living beyond that age and a 50% chance of dying before that age. Since you can't be sure which will apply to you, assume you'll live at least a few years past the average. Consider your present health as well as how long other family members have lived.

RATE OF RETURN

A few decades ago, many retirement plans were calculated using fairly high rates of return. At a minimum, make sure your expectations are based on average returns over an extended period. You might even want to be more conservative, assuming a rate of return lower than long-term averages suggest. Even a small difference in your estimated and actual rate of return can make a significant difference in your ultimate savings.

INFLATION

Even modest levels of inflation can significantly affect the purchasing power of your money over long time periods. For instance, after 30 years of just 2% inflation, your portfolio's purchasing power will decline by 45%. When estimating an inflation figure, don't just look at the historically low inflation rates from the recent past; also consider long-term inflation rates, since your retirement could last for decades.

RETIREMENT TAX RATE

If you save large amounts in tax-deferred investments that will be taxable when withdrawn, your tax rate can significantly affect the amount you'll have available for spending. You may find your tax rate is the same or higher after retirement.

As you can see, there is no simple or universal answer to the retirement feasibility question. Your financial advisor should be able to assist you in choosing the direction needed to attain the ultimate goal of a successful retirement.

SMART PLANNING

Physicians contemplating retirement within a few years need to understand the future risks of the financial situation they may be facing. People are living longer, which means you may have to provide for a bigger cushion in retirement than you initially intended. In addition, uncertainty over future Social Security benefits as Baby Boomers continue to retire adds to the concerns. As a result, you could face a personal shortfall, especially if you incur unforeseen expenses from a medical condition or other situation.

So, what could/should you do? Even if retirement is imminent, you may be able to make up lost ground quickly or take other steps to protect yourself. Here are several ideas to consider:

- Maximize retirement savings vehicles. Just a few years of making contributions at or near the maximum level can significantly bolster your account. If you have qualified retirement plans that you are not fully funding, determine if your cash flow will allow you to do so.
- Work on the budget. This tool was important when you started your career, but it is critical now. If an analysis of financial planning for retirement determines that you may have a potential shortfall, consider dialing down your expectations. Make realistic estimates about future income you expect and potential expenses. Although you likely will be paying less for housing and other items such as life insurance, especially if your children are adults, consider the impact of potential increases in such expenses as travel.
- Move to a smaller home or condo: For most people, housing is the largest overall cost, representing on average more than one-third of overall spending.

If your kids no longer live with you, but you're still living in the large home where you raised them, it may be time to downsize. In addition, you might want to move to a state with a different climate, or a state with lower taxes. Of course, other factors such as proximity to family and personal preferences will come into play.

- Refinance your current home. If you decide not to downsize, consider refinancing an existing mortgage if you are paying a rate higher than those currently available. At the beginning of 2013, mortgage rates had reached historic lows. Even though rates have increased slightly since then, you may save tens of thousands of dollars over time by refinancing. Keep in mind that your interest payments will generally continue to be tax-deductible.

- Do not stop working altogether. Just because you have reached retirement age does not mean you have to stop working completely. If necessary, pursue part-time employment. For some individuals, working full-time a little longer is also a viable option. (We have provided you with options for continuing working or being engaged in some healthcare capacity in Chapter 13.)

Every physician's situation is unique, but the most important thing to do is assess your financial planning objectives, including a review of your investment portfolio. Planning involves assumptions about the future—assumptions that may not pan out. Although you cannot avoid making assumptions, you can evaluate whether they are realistic and consider how your lifestyle might change if future economic and financial conditions are much different than projected. And while you also cannot fully control the factors involved in portfolio endurance during retirement, having more wealth can improve the odds of having a less stressful financial life. A more substantial nest egg might enable you to take fewer risks, enjoy a higher sustainable lifestyle, or extend the productive life of your portfolio.

INDIVIDUAL RETIREMENT ACCOUNTS

Often times we are so focused on the benefits of *contributing* to a retirement plan or Individual Retirement Account (IRA) that we forget about eventually having to address *distributing* what we've accumulated. What many retirees don't realize is that the IRS not only limits the amount you can contribute to qualified retirement plans and IRAs while you are working, it decides how much you must withdraw when you're retired. Under the rules for "required minimum distributions" (RMDs), you may have to take distributions before the end of the year, whether you want to or not.

First, know that distributions from qualified retirement plans and IRAs are taxed at ordinary income rates. In addition, you must pay a 10% penalty tax on distributions received prior to age 59½, unless a special exception applies (IRC

Section 72t). On the other hand, RMDs are not required for Roth IRAs based on current tax law.

Usually you must begin taking RMDs no later than April 1 of the year following the year in which you reach age 70½. For example, if you are turning age 70½ this year, the first distribution must occur by April 1 next year. But if you wait that long, you will also have to take another distribution for that year by December 31. To avoid the doubling up of payouts in one year, you can arrange to take your payout prior to April 1 of the year after you turn 70½. Once you pass age 70½, you must continue taking annual distributions.

However, there is an exception to these rules if you still work on a full-time basis and you do not own 5% or more of your practice or other business entity. In this case, you are allowed to postpone RMDs until your actual retirement.

How much do you have to withdraw? The amount of the annual RMD is based on the IRS life expectancy tables for the age you will attain in the current year and the value of the account on the last day of the previous calendar year. In other words, your RMD for the current tax year depends on the age you will attain in the current year and your balance as of December 31 of the previous year, even though you're taking out the funds almost a full year later. Your financial advisor or tax advisor can help you determine the amount of your specific required distributions. In addition, there are many websites that have RMD calculators to use on your own.

If you fail to comply with these rules, the IRS may impose a harsh penalty equal to 50% of the amount that should have been withdrawn, or the difference between the required amount and a lesser amount actually withdrawn. The penalty is added to the regular income tax that is due on the RMD. To avoid any potential problems, be sure to take your distributions well in advance of the December 31 deadline. Don't wait until the last moment.

The key is to be proactive and plan accordingly. So often, the vast majority of time is spent on determining the best way to shelter income through various qualified retirement plans, and very little attention is paid to the rules for taking the money out. Keep in mind that during your retirement years, you will have two separate pools of assets to draw from: qualified (retirement plans and IRAs) and non-qualified (personal investment portfolios). By utilizing distributions from both sources, you can create an income stream during retirement that minimizes income taxation, avoids penalties, and maximizes the efficiencies within your overall coordinated financial plan.

Post-retirement rollover IRAs (IRA/RO) generally represent most physicians' largest financial asset. With this is mind, ensure that your retirement account beneficiary decisions are made carefully. While many institutions provide custody services for traditional IRA assets, the onus is on the IRA owner to make the ultimate beneficiary decision. Unfortunately, many physicians don't take the time to understand and personally individualize the beneficiary language within the agreement to meet their specific objectives. Understanding the impact that the beneficiary designation has on the distribution of the account after the IRA owner dies is a critical element of the planning process.

From the standpoint of those who inherit a traditional contributory IRA or IRA/RO (as opposed to a Roth IRA), it's important to understand the unique rules associated with the process, which is different for spousal beneficiaries and non-spouse beneficiaries.

If you are the sole beneficiary of your spouse's traditional IRA, you may choose to treat that IRA as your own. This means you can contribute to the IRA if you are eligible to do so, and, if you are younger than 70½, you do not have to take RMDs. As an alternative, you may leave the IRA in your spouse's name with you as the beneficiary. If your deceased spouse died after age 70½, you generally must base subsequent RMDs on the longer of your single life expectancy or the deceased's life expectancy. Otherwise, distributions may be based on your single life expectancy or the account must be totally liquidated in five years. Another possible option is to roll over the inherited IRA assets into your own IRA. The rollover is exempt from current tax liability if completed within 60 days.

If, on the other hand, you inherit an IRA from someone other than your spouse, you cannot treat the IRA as your own. Thus, you are not allowed to make subsequent contributions to the inherited IRA nor can you roll over the funds to your own IRA. You must begin taking RMDs subject to the rules for IRA beneficiaries. Distributions from an inherited IRA are taxed as ordinary income. If you fail to take an RMD, you must pay a penalty equal to 50% of the required amount of the distribution.

Married IRA owners usually name their spouse as beneficiary and either do not name a contingent beneficiary or give very little consideration to whom to name. Those who do name a contingent beneficiary often name their children. In that case, caution does need to be exercised in the event that one of the named children dies prior to the IRA owner. Typically, the deceased child's portion of the inheritance would go to the other living children, as opposed to the deceased child's family. This may indeed be your objective. However, if your intention is to have your child's portion pass through to his or her heirs, be sure to add the line: "to my descendants per stirpes." The Latin term "per stirpes" means "by right of the deceased." This specific legal terminology will ensure that if the beneficiary child dies, his or her descendants get the full share.

There are many IRA intricacies and nuances that you should address to ensure you are maximizing both income tax and estate tax planning opportunities. Be sure to consult with your tax or financial advisor to ensure your IRA is structured properly now in order to avoid surprises or problems for your heirs in the future.

SOCIAL SECURITY BENEFITS

As you approach retirement, one of the key decisions you will face is when to begin receiving Social Security benefits. It is not an easy call, and the answer usually depends on your personal circumstances. The sliding scale used to calculate benefits, which pays a smaller monthly check if you retire "early" and more if you wait longer, depends on the year you were born. Your lifetime payout depends on how long you live. The first step is to visit www.ssa.gov/planners/calculators.htm1 and find out when you're entitled to full benefits and how much those benefits are.

Keeping your projected benefits in mind, the Social Security Administration (SSA) provides three basic timeframes to consider for planning purposes: early retirement, normal or "full" retirement, and late retirement.

- Early retirement: You are eligible to begin receiving Social Security retiree benefits as early as age 62. However, you will receive a reduced benefit if you retire before you reach your full retirement age. For example, if you retire at age 62, your benefit will be about 25% lower than if you waited for full retirement age.
- Normal (full) retirement: The age at which you can begin receiving full retirement benefits depends on when you were born. If you were born in 1948 or earlier, you are already eligible for full Social Security benefits. If you were born between 1943 and 1960, the age for receiving full retirement benefits gradually increases to age 67.
- Late retirement: You may choose to keep working beyond the normal retirement age to receive greater retirement benefits or delay your application for retirement benefits. If you are considering late retirement, keep in mind that each additional year you work adds another year of earnings to your Social Security record. Higher lifetime earnings may provide greater benefits to you in retirement. In addition, your benefit will increase automatically by a certain percentage from the time you reach your full retirement age until you start receiving your benefits or until you reach age 70. The percentage varies depending on your year of birth. For example, someone who reaches full retirement age (66) qualifies for an annual Social Security benefit of $30,420. However, if this individual delays the start of benefit until age 70, the benefit increases to $40,154—an increase of nearly 32%.

The Social Security benefit timing decision gets a bit complicated if you expect to claim benefits based on your spouse's earning record. Typically, a spouse who has not worked, or one who has had low earnings, may receive up to one-half of the other spouse's full benefit. If you are eligible to receive both your own retirement benefits and spousal benefits, your own benefits are paid out first. However, if your benefits as a spouse would exceed your own retirement benefits, you may receive a combination of benefits equaling the higher benefit.

Once you have reached your full retirement age, you may choose to receive only your spouse's benefits. In that case, you will continue accruing delayed retirement credits on your own Social Security record. Then you may file for benefits at a later date, up to age 70, and receive a higher monthly benefit based on the delayed retirement credits.

Other special rules may apply for widows and widowers, divorced spouses, and those entitled to receive disability benefits. You can find more information on these topics by visiting the SSA website at *www.ssa.gov*.

Ultimately, regardless of the timing option, because payments are based on your projected expected life expectancy, which in reality is an unknown, your decision will likely have to be fully coordinated with your overall personal retirement and financial plan.

LIFE INSURANCE

If you have sufficient investment assets to meet your survivor income objectives, do you still need life insurance?

Consider why life insurance is purchased in the first place. People buy life insurance when they do not have sufficient assets to provide for their survivors. If you have sufficient assets, then you are considered to be self-insured. In many instances, a physician's greatest need for life insurance is early in their career, prior to having accumulated substantial assets. There are many different types of life insurance products available to meet the varying needs of physicians. The key, regardless of the reason you are buying life insurance, is to be certain that the specific life insurance product you are purchasing meets your unique objectives.

The starting point in any life insurance planning exercise is deciding on the amount and type of coverage needed. What you bought early in your career may not be the optimal coverage for you as you approach retirement or are completely retired. Do you still need life insurance during retirement? Each situation is different. Begin by determining if you still have a need, and if so, is your specific life insurance need temporary or permanent. Temporary would imply that your needs are relatively short-term. A good example would be if you are trying to provide survivor income in the event you die prior to becoming self-insured. Permanent insurance, on the other hand, is generally purchased with the understanding that the policy proceeds will be paid out at the time of your death, regardless of when that occurs, even if you live beyond your expected mortality age.

Many physicians recognize the benefits of an overall financial plan to meet their long-term objectives such as retirement planning, education planning, and investment planning. However, planning for the unexpected, via life insurance, is certainly less pleasant and may be difficult. Understandably, no one likes to contemplate their own demise, and there are so many other important issues that seem to take precedence over the life insurance decision making process. Whatever the reason, delaying this important part of the financial planning process can result in expensive and unintended tragic consequences. When planning for survivor income needs, consider the ongoing income needs of your survivors, as well as any immediate lump sum needs. Once you have defined the qualitative and quantitative need for life insurance, you can determine which specific product in the life insurance marketplace best meets your objectives.

The life insurance decision does not end there, however. It is necessary to consider the intricacies of how death benefits pass to the intended heirs, and how your estate is impacted, prior to purchasing a policy. Specifically, give careful consideration as to who should be the owner of the policy. While insurance proceeds aren't subject to income taxes, they can be subject to estate taxes. The four most common ways to own a life insurance policy are:

1. By the insured. If you own the policy, the insurance proceeds will be considered part of your taxable estate and may be subject to estate taxes if your estate is large enough.
2. By the insured's spouse. The insurance proceeds won't be included in your taxable estate if your spouse both owns the policy and is the beneficiary of the policy, unless you inherit the policy under the terms of your spouse's will. However, if someone else is named as beneficiary, such as a child, the proceeds will be considered a gift and may be subject to gift taxes.
3. By a person other than the insured's spouse. In this situation, the insurance proceeds won't be included in your taxable estate. However, keep in mind that if you want to pay the insurance premiums, premiums in excess of $14,000 for 2016 (unchanged from 2015) may be considered taxable gifts. In situations where you have two or more beneficiaries, you will have to gift the money for the premiums to the beneficiaries in order to qualify for the gift tax exclusion.

Minor children can't own insurance policies in most states, so you may have to set up a custodial account if the owners are minors. Care must be taken if you are transferring an existing policy—this is considered a gift, which may trigger gift taxes if the cash value exceeds $14,000. Also, if you die within three years of transferring a policy, the proceeds will still be included in your taxable estate.

4. By a trust. When a trust owns the policy, the proceeds are not considered part of your taxable estate if the trust is irrevocable and you are not the beneficiary, meaning that you can't change the terms or terminate the trust. The same tax rules apply to trusts as those applicable to a person other than your spouse, but you often can structure more flexibility into a trust arrangement.

5. While it may seem easiest to simply own the policy and have a spouse be the beneficiary, as you can see, other options may be more favorable. Spend some time with your financial planner to determine the most efficient way to structure your life insurance policies. Only in this manner will your insurance plan be properly coordinated with your overall financial plan in an effort to minimize or reduce estate taxation.

BYPASS TRUSTS

Successful estate planning generally involves passing your assets on to your heirs with minimal tax consequences. Bypass trusts, which are sometimes called credit shelter trusts, are set up by married couples to minimize estate taxes. The main advantage of a bypass trust is that the assets used to fund the trust are not included in either spouse's taxable estate for federal estate tax purposes. Typically, a bypass trust is funded with assets that have a value equal to no more than the current federal estate tax exemption amount. The bypass trust is funded when the first spouse passes away. Since the objective is to "bypass" the taxable estates of both spouses, the best assets to use for funding bypass trusts are those that are expected to appreciate. That way, any future appreciation will not be subject to estate taxes, even after the death of the second spouse.

However, when a bypass trust is designated as the beneficiary of a tax-favored retirement account, the account generally must be liquidated under the RMD rules over the life expectancy of the oldest bypass trust beneficiary. In other words, the RMD rules turn the account into a depreciating asset. What if the retirement account owner's estate is designated as the account beneficiary and the account is then used to fund a bypass trust under the terms of the account owner's will? In that case, the account generally must be liquidated over an even shorter period under the required minimum distribution rules.

Taxable savings vehicles that contain assets expected to appreciate, such as stocks and equity mutual funds, are good candidates for funding bypass trusts for two primary reasons:

1. Funding the bypass trust with appreciating assets allows the future appreciation to escape estate tax for either spouse.
2. The cost basis (for income tax purposes) of capital gain assets used to fund a bypass trust will be stepped up to fair market value as of the date of the account owner's death. So the bypass trust will have a stepped-up tax basis in the assets, which will reduce or eliminate the capital gains tax when they are later sold.

What about funding a bypass trust with taxable accounts that are loaded with cash equivalents and fixed income assets? They are only adequate candidates because they are also not appreciating assets. However, they are preferable to tax-favored retirement accounts. Your estate planning advisor can help you plan a trust that contains the best assets for tax minimization purposes.

REAL PROPERTY

There are many ways you can hold title to real property, which is defined as land and anything built on it. However, the way in which real property is titled will affect how it is transferred during the administration of an estate, so understanding the differences is important.

Subject to the terminology of each state, most people who own private residences are:

- Sole owners;
- Joint owners with rights of survivorship (the property is owned with another person and either party can inherit the other party's share);
- Tenants in common (an individual owns property with another person but the heirs of each party inherit their own share);
- Tenants by the entirety (a married couple owns property with each spouse passing it to the surviving spouse); or
- Through an entity such as a corporation, LLC, or partnership.

Each ownership situation must be dealt with during the estate administration process. Make sure you own real estate in a way that will fulfill your wishes upon death and, at the same time, streamline the process of transferring ownership of the property. Estate planning techniques to avoid probate depend on how you choose to hold title to the property. The most common way to avoid probate is for spouses to own property as tenants by the entirety. By owning the property together, it passes to the surviving spouse outside of the probate process, avoiding delays.

Another way to avoid probate is for two individuals to own the real property jointly with rights of survivorship. However, you must be careful that this option meets your wishes because you may not want the other owner to inherit your share of the property when considering the total value of your estate as a whole.

Still another way to own real property that allows for the avoidance of probate is with a revocable living trust. The benefit of the trust holding title to the real estate is that the trust document specifically addresses who will inherit the property without having the need to probate the property.

If a property you own has a mortgage and you want to place it in a trust, there are additional considerations. You must review the mortgage agreement and, in most cases, get pre-approval of the transfer of property. Generally though, mortgage companies permit the transfer to a revocable trust. Some owners of real property want to avoid personal liability, especially if they own commercial or rental property. These owners typically create a corporation or a limited liability company (LLC) to own the real property. This provides some protection from being personally responsible for the debts or liabilities of the entity. At the time of death, these shares or membership interests in the corporation or LLC pass through the individual's estate through the probate process. In the individual's will, the testator (the person whose will it is) can designate who will inherit the share of the corporation, or allow it to pass to the residual estate.

Holding title as tenants in common will result in the property going through probate and sometimes results in contention with the other owner and the persons who will inherit your share or the other party's share. It is best to discuss these issues with the other owner and the heirs to help alleviate any tension that may occur in the future with new ownership of the real property.

Consult your estate planning advisor about the best way to hold your real property so that you have an estate plan that best meets your wishes and streamlines the transfer process.

A MATTER OF TAXES

While the American Taxpayer Relief Act of 2012 (ATRA) provides relatively generous estate tax rates, limits, and rules for estates, that doesn't mean estate planning in general should fall from your radar.

Specifically, the ATRA reduced the top marginal federal estate tax rate from 55% to 40%, increased the federal estate tax exemption from $1 million to $5 million (adjusted annually for inflation) and made portability of the estate tax exemption permanent. The federal estate tax exemption is $5.45 million for 2016—and it will go even higher in future years if it continues to be indexed to inflation.

As a result, in most cases, estate planning for federal tax purposes now focuses on increasing the tax basis of transferred assets, reducing capital gains on asset sales, and taking advantage of capital losses while you're still alive.

If you continue to own appreciated capital assets (such as stocks, mutual fund shares, real estate and collectibles) until you or your spouse dies, the tax consequence could be greatly reduced, or even completely eliminated, when the assets are eventually sold. This taxpayer-friendly outcome is courtesy of Section 1014(a) of the Internal Revenue Code which generally allows an unlimited federal income tax basis step-up for appreciated capital assets owned by a person who passes away.

Under this rule, the income tax basis of appreciated capital assets, including personal residences, are stepped up to fair market value (FMV) as of the date of death (or the alternate valuation date six months later, if applicable). When the value of an asset eligible for this favorable rule stays about the same between the date of death and the date of sale by the decedent's heirs, there will be little or no taxable gain to report to the IRS. That's because the sales proceeds will be fully offset (or nearly so) by the stepped-up basis.

If you are married and your spouse predeceases you, the basis of the portion of the home owned by your spouse, typically 50%, gets stepped up to FMV. This usually removes half of the appreciation that has occurred over the years from the federal income tax return. If you continue to own the home until you die, the basis in the part you own at that point, which will usually be 100%, gets stepped up to FMV as of the date of your death (or six months later, if applicable). So, your heirs can subsequently sell the property and owe little or no federal tax on the sale.

While hanging onto appreciated capital assets can be a tax-smart strategy, the opposite is true for depreciated capital assets (those with current FMV below cost). If these assets are sold, capital losses are triggered. They can be used to shelter capital gains from selling appreciated assets. However, if a depreciated capital asset is held until death, the tax basis will be reduced to the lower current FMV. If the asset is then sold by the estate or an heir, there won't be any tax-saving capital loss.

Individuals should also consider giving appreciated capital assets (such as stock and mutual fund shares) to IRS-approved charities. The tax-saving advantage is that you can generally claim an itemized charitable donation deduction equal to the current FMV of the appreciated asset while also avoiding any capital gains tax on the appreciation.

Estate planning is a continuous process that should be reviewed on a regular basis to ensure you're aware of the latest trends.

GIFTS AND CHARITABLE CONTRIBUTIONS

There are a number of reasons to give to charitable causes. From a purely financial standpoint, gifts to a charity during lifetime or at death will reduce the size of the gross estate, which may reduce or even eliminate the estate taxes at death. An additional benefit of lifetime gifts is that a current income tax deduction is available within certain percentage limitations.

If the estate owner, based on his or her current financial situation, is not willing or able to contribute an entire financial asset during his or her lifetime, he or she may consider a split interest, deferred gift. The ownership interests in an asset can be split or divided into two parts, a stream of income payable for one or more lifetimes, or a term of years (the income interest) and the principal remaining after the income term (the remainder interest). When the estate owner retains the right to the income but transfers his or her rights in the remainder to a trust, it is called a charitable remainder trust.

To qualify for an income tax deduction, the trust must be a unitrust, an annuity trust, a pooled income fund, or a charitable gift annuity.

- Charitable remainder unitrust. In this type of trust, the donor retains the right to a fixed percentage of the FMV of the trust assets, with the trust assets being re-valued annually. If the value of the assets increases, so does the annual payout, and vice versa.
- Charitable remainder annuity trust. This trust is similar to the unitrust but pays a fixed dollar amount each year.
- Pooled income fund. Assets are transferred to a common investment fund maintained by the charity. Each donor receives a share of the income from the fund annually, in proportion to the contribution made. These annual payments continue for the life of the donor and spouse. At death, the corpus of the donor's gift, together with any capital gains, passes to the charity. Payments will increase or decrease with the investment performance of the fund.
- Charitable gift annuity. The donor transfers the asset directly to the charity in exchange for the charity's agreement to pay a fixed lifetime annuity.

The amount of the income tax deduction depends on the percentage of the income interest and the period over which it will be paid (usually the life of the donor and his or her spouse). This calculation is determined from the mortality tables published by the federal government.

On the other end of the charitable gifting spectrum are those individuals who want the charity to receive only the income and not the asset itself. A charitable income or lead trust is the reverse of the charitable remainder trust. The income interest is assigned to the charity, usually for a period of years, and the remainder generally passes to the donor's heirs. The amount of the estate tax deduction and the amount left for the heirs depends on the number of years of income to be paid to the charity, the size of the annual payments, and the investment results achieved by the trustee.

There are many factors to consider prior to implementing any type of charitable trust strategy. To determine if it makes sense for your particular situation, consult with your tax and estate planning advisors.

TRUSTS

Trusts are frequently used in estate planning to manage assets as well as minimize probate expenses and estate taxes. Despite their apparent complexity, trusts can be useful in many aspects of planning your estate.

Before you begin discussions with an estate planning attorney, you need to understand the various roles of the parties affiliated with the trust.

- The grantor is the individual who transfers funds into the trust.
- The trustee makes certain the terms of the trust, as outlined by the grantor, are carried out.
- The beneficiary is the individual (or individuals) for whom the trust has been created. Often a minor, the beneficiary can also be a surviving spouse, adult child, or any individual in need of financial assistance (or supervision) after the death of the grantor.

You can now focus on the different types of basic trusts most often used for estate planning purposes.

Testamentary trust. This trust is usually part of a will and comes into existence after death. With a testamentary trust, assets are passed through probate before being managed by the trust. The trust can then help divide assets for each beneficiary, manage assets, or distribute assets as required by the directions of the trust.

Living trust or inter-vivos trust. Basically, this trust is created during the life of the grantor; assets are transferred into the trust and will thus avoid probate at the time of death. As an added benefit, living trusts provide benefits during life, particularly in the event of the incompetency of the grantor. A living trust identifies a list of contingent trustees who are able to assume the managerial responsibilities of the trust in the event the original trustee (usually the grantor) is unable to perform his or her duties. Such forethought avoids the excessive legal costs involved if a grantor is declared incompetent, since in such cases, annual accountings to the court are required.

A trust can be an effective way to control the management and distribution of assets. However, a trust only works to the extent that assets have been transferred into the trust. Often times, physicians spend hours in their attorneys' offices creating what they hope will be the perfect trust arrangement for their estate. Unfortunately, many never get around to transferring their assets into the trust. If you create a trust for your estate plan, make certain your assets are titled in the way necessary for the trust to work, since asset titling and beneficiary designations take precedence over the directives of your will or trust.

For example, if you have a large life insurance policy naming your surviving spouse as beneficiary, a residence and summer home jointly titled with your spouse, and various investment accounts also jointly titled with your spouse, all of that will pass directly to your spouse, bypassing any trust arrangement you paid to put in place. Whatever plans the survivor has made (or may make) will be the controlling factor for all assets going forward.

To control the distribution and management of the assets, to minimize estate tax liability and ultimately probate expenses, it is necessary to revisit all titling and beneficiary designations. Your estate planning attorney, working in tandem with your investment and insurance advisors, can assist in this process to ensure a well-coordinated and effective estate plan.

NUTS AND BOLTS OF PLANNING

Few physicians view estate planning as an urgent or immediate need. In fact, most physicians initiate their estate plan prior to traveling abroad or from their deathbed. This approach is to be avoided at all costs. Without a properly structured estate plan, your heirs may pay unnecessary estate taxes and probate fees that in many cases can be dramatically reduced or even eliminated with careful planning.

While financial planners can help determine the various goals, objectives, and actual structure of the estate plan, you ultimately will need to engage the services of a qualified estate planning attorney in order to draft and implement your plan. Because attorneys bill for their time, being well-prepared prior to the initial meeting can save substantial time, which translates to lower legal fees.

Several decisions should be made prior to meeting with the attorney who will be drafting the estate planning documents. For individuals with minor children, perhaps one of the most important and difficult decisions relates to choosing a guardian. While your heart may tell you to select grandparents, be mindful of their age and ability to raise another family. Other options may include a sibling or a close friend. Factors to consider include: ages of the proposed guardians and the ages of their children, ages of your children, and the health and financial situation of all parties. It is also an excellent idea to decide on alternative choices in the event your first choice is unwilling or unable to serve. If you name a married couple as guardians and one of them dies or the couple divorces, consider whether you want one of them to act as the sole guardian.

You must also select an executor for your estate. It is the executor's responsibility, via the probate process, to handle the details of paying any debts of the estate as well as death taxes, and distributing the remaining assets to the beneficiaries named in your will.

Prior to meeting with the attorney, make a list of all of your assets, including their values as well as how each asset is owned, either individually or jointly titled. This will give the attorney a snapshot of the value of your estate as well as the level of probate exposure.

If you are going to use various trust strategies, you will need to name a trustee to manage investments and take care of issues relating to the trust, such as the various types of distributions that will be made. The trustee can be an individual or a corporate fiduciary such as a bank trust company.

Another decision deals with the ages of your children at the time the estate is distributed. If you do not want to distribute assets to your children outright, in a lump sum, upon your and/or your spouse's death, the assets can be held in trust for their benefit. And, the ultimate distribution does not have to be made as a lump sum. Many prefer to make distributions of a portion of the estate at several different times; e.g., 1/3 at age 21, 1/3 at age 25, and 1/3 at age 30, or any other combination you believe works best for your children.

Lastly, you will need to make arrangements in the event your children predecease the distribution of the estate. Decisions need to be made today as to whom the ultimate beneficiaries will be if this were to happen—other relatives, friends, or even charity.

While these issues are difficult and emotionally taxing to address, planning ahead will eliminate wasted time sitting in the attorney's office with the money clock ticking away.

FINAL INSTRUCTIONS

Estate planning encompasses a multitude of strategies and techniques to reduce estate taxation and ultimately pass property to heirs. Often forgotten in the process, however, is the need to prepare a letter of final instruction.

A letter of final instruction provides an informal personal inventory that is not legally binding. Typically, the letter is addressed to a surviving spouse, adult children, lawyers, or to the executor. The goal is to ensure that those closest to you are aware of the assets that otherwise might prove difficult or even impossible to find upon your death or serious injury. Additionally, instructions can be included pertaining to funeral arrangements or any other issues that may require direction, including the exact location of all important papers needed to settle the estate.

The letter of final instruction can also serve as an informal will, specifying which beneficiaries will receive certain assets. It may inform others of certain benefits of which they may not be aware. The following items should be included:

- List of all potential fringe benefits due to the heirs from your practice or employer, including life or accident insurance benefits;
- Detail of any expected benefits from Social Security or other government services such as veterans benefits; and
- List of all retirement plans, including 401k, profit sharing, pension plans, and IRAs.

Be sure to list the names, addresses, and telephone numbers of people and organizations to notify in the event of your death. This list may include relatives, friends, clergy, attorneys, accountants, investment managers, insurance agents, financial institutions, and colleagues.

It is also important to indicate the exact location of important documents, specifically wills, trusts, birth and marriage certificates, divorce agreements, title to property such as homes and automobiles, and any other legal papers. There should also be a listing of all bank and investment account numbers and the location of documents such as savings account passbooks and checks. It is also a good idea to describe where old tax returns, investment confirmations, and credit card statements can be found.

If you maintain a safe deposit box, record the contents and location of the boxes, a list of those who have access to the safe deposit box, and where the keys to the box are kept.

A letter of final instruction can even provide you with the opportunity to write your own obituary or simply indicate what you would want mentioned in it, including charitable entities to which you may want to direct donations. The same also applies to funeral arrangements. The letter can be used to instruct others as to how simple or elaborate a funeral you want to have and whether you have already bought a cemetery plot and made arrangements with a specific funeral home.

Unlike a will, which becomes binding at the time of death, this letter is not legally binding. But this may also prove advantageous since you easily are able to make any changes that you want at any time prior to death. Attach a copy to your will, send one to your lawyer or executor, and keep one at home, in a place where your family will know to find it.

SUMMARY

You have worked hard during your training and career, and now is the time to settle into your next stage of life. From a financial planning perspective, the focus shifts from accumulating assets to determining how to best use your financial resources to provide income. This time of life also allows you to reexamine the strategies you have used and determine if changes need to be made based on your new requirements.

It's important to realize that financial planning evolves over time, and often times changes need to be made as various goals are met and new goals emerge. If successful, you can now reap the benefits of all of the earlier planning and saving you did while working in your medical career. One of the greatest benefits of diligent lifetime planning is the peace of mind associated with knowing that you are doing everything possible to ensure a successful retirement, as well as ensuring an efficient passing of your wealth based on your wishes and tax efficiency. Congratulations!

CHAPTER 16

Deciding What Comes Next: Enjoying Life After Practice

Peter S. Moskowitz, MD and Neil H. Baum, MD

*"Half our life is spent trying to find something to do with
the time we have rushed through life trying to save."*

Will Rogers

A S PHYSICIANS, WE LEAD VERY structured lives. We wake up at a designated time, report to the hospital, the operating room, the clinic at a designated time, take care of patients again over a specified time, and then finish up with returning phone calls, completing paperwork, or doing obligatory journal reading at our desks or at our bedside. Evenings are spent planning for the next day, answering emails, and staying abreast of the latest developments in our areas of interest or expertise.

Contrast this with retirement: no specific time to wake up in the morning; no place to be at a time when others are waiting for us; no committee meetings to attend; no staff to hire, fire, or motivate; no paperwork to complete; and no journals that must be read. Is it any wonder that physicians become disoriented with the new lifestyle?

In Chapter 14, we presented the rationale to begin retirement planning early in a doctor's career— "protirement." As you will recall, that term refers to the proactive process of retirement planning, including a vision for your retirement years, a financial plan and income plan for retirement, and detailed considerations for how you will have fun, connect with others, and find meaning and contribution after closing your practice.

Prior chapters have provided roadmaps for selling your practice and the basic principles of getting to financial independence. In this chapter, the assumption is that you have been conscientious about your protirement planning and have reached the glorious last day of clinical practice. We will now focus on reaping the benefits of your many hard years of work and your diligent planning for your retirement years.

Now it is time to implement your protirement plan!

STAYING HEALTHY AND HAPPY IN RETIREMENT

Staying healthy has to become the basis of your retirement success and happiness. During the many long years of a demanding medical career, most physicians did not consistently take good care of themselves physically, emotionally, or spiritually. Now in retirement, we have no excuses not to do that. Without your health, you have nothing.

Chapter 13 provided general guidelines for developing and sustaining physical fitness. What follows here are some brief suggestions to guide your thinking and actions regarding sustaining good health.

Institute Personal Wellness

We all know the meaning of these two words. Develop a written, well-thought-out plan to get healthier than you have ever been. That plan should include aerobic physical activity at least three days a week, healthy eating, sleeping at least seven to eight hours nightly, and active intellectual pursuits. You should have an annual physical exam and your entire wellness program should be monitored by a physician other than you.

Build Self-Awareness

Self-awareness is important for emotional balance and emotional intelligence. Some easy strategies for self-awareness include spending five minutes a day in quiet solitude, writing in a personal journal daily, regular prayer, and meditation.

Utilize Values-Based Management of Your Time and Your Money

Doctors often "overspend" their available time and their money. By that, we mean that we allow our plate to get too full, we have a hard time saying "no," and in so doing become over-committed. That leads to stress or worse. The meaning of overspending our money is self-evident. Becoming over-burdened with credit card debt or other indebtedness is a second powerful form of stress. As a part of protirement discussed in Chapter 14, physicians should strive to clarify how they want to allocate their time in retirement and how they wish to allocate their income in retirement. Then, stick to your plan. Get professional help, when necessary, to keep yourself accountable and on track.

Stay Connected to a Community(s) and Family

All humans thrive through connection to others. The one danger of retirement is that it is relatively easy to become isolated after we leave our familiar practice environments. Spend time with your family and loved ones—that goes without saying. Spoil your grandchildren, learn from them how to have spontaneous fun. Find groups of people outside of your family and loved ones who share your interests, hobbies, favorite sports, political interests, and so forth. These people become your communities. Spend time regularly with your communities. Have fun and share your life with these people. The more communities in your life, the happier you will be in retirement.

Save Time for Daily Fun

Many of us were so intent in being the best physician we could be that we eventually forgot how to have fun. Rediscover fun in retirement. If you don't know how, find a friend who is full of fun and take some lessons. Engage your spouse, engage your children and grandchildren. Take a risk and learn some new game or outdoor activity. Most importantly, find a little time each and every day for fun. You will live longer and happier.

Balance Your Life

Work-life balance is the most potent form of managing your stress and preventing professional burnout. In retirement, it sustains happiness, health, and a sense of well-being. Review the six domains of balance and strategies for sustaining balance provided in Chapter 7.

Repair Relationships That Need Improvement

No one goes through a long life without some relationship mishaps. Unfortunately, many of those mishaps involve people we are closest to: our spouse, our children, our parents, our professional partners. Holding onto anger and resentment is toxic to your emotional and physical health and your happiness. Strive to make amends where necessary. Apologize when it is appropriate. All that is required is some humility. Love and forgiveness make the world a better place. Life is too short; repair your relationships in retirement.

Expand Your Friendships

Overwhelmingly, most physicians' answer to the question, "how many intimate friends do you have?" is "none" or "one." While in active clinical practice, most physicians simply don't have the time or the energy to sustain intimate friendships. When they do have close friends, they are almost always other physicians.

Retirement provides an opportunity to do things differently, a time to stop being socially isolated or lonely. Find ways to meet new people, get engaged in new activities, volunteer your time, become active in your church, mosque, or synagogue. Doing so will enrich your life with vibrant and stimulating new friendships.

Challenge Your Intellect

Physicians and physicians-in-training discover very quickly that medical science changes so rapidly that in order to stay current, they must practice continuous learning throughout their career. It is a tribute to the profession that physicians do this so successfully and consistently. In retirement, the incentive to continue to study so diligently is less intense, yet the need for intellectual stimulation remains strong.

In addition to reading your favorite medical resources in retirement, find new ways to challenge your mind. Read books from the bestseller list, join a book club and read a book a month, take a course at your local community college, university, or an online course, on topics that interest you. Learn more about managing your retirement investment portfolio or how to do those home repair projects you have been putting off for years. Keeping your mind active and challenged has been shown to prolong your life and reduce the incidence of dementia.

Give Away Your Personal Gifts

We are all born with a unique set of skills and gifts that set us apart from others. These gifts are largely responsible for our personal and professional success in life. One way to sustain happiness in retirement is to give away our gifts to others. Volunteering, mentoring others, teaching, spending time with people less advantaged are all good ways to give away your gifts.

WHAT DO YOU WANT TO DO IN RETIREMENT?

Perhaps writing about what to do in retirement is superfluous. After all, you've been thinking and dreaming about it for years before the actual day arrives. Nevertheless, we will draw from our own retirement experience and that of many physician clients whose experience in retirement offers some interesting perspectives.

Travel

Travel can be one of your greatest pleasures—experiencing cultures in other parts of the world that are substantially different from your own. The more adventurous, the better. Travel need not be to the far corners of the planet; two or three days away from your home and your usual routine can do wonders to brighten your mood and outlook. For many physicians, travel offers the first real opportunity to explore the world because they could rarely get more than a week away from the practice.

Volunteer

A strong desire to help others and make the world a better place are reasons cited by many physicians as their motivation to enter medicine. In retirement, those same basic motivators are still typically present. Many retired physicians find great satisfaction and meaning by volunteering their skills and experience in any one of hundreds of different public and private institutions, business, schools, clinics, programs for the needy anywhere in the world.

If personal fulfillment is the primary concern and finances are not an issue, many physicians find volunteer projects or charitable endeavors to keep busy. Volunteer work can be very rewarding, and giving back will help fulfill the need to make a difference or to be useful in a fashion as helping our patients lead healthy lifestyles. Many physicians who don't need to return to work for financial reasons simply want to give back to the community and serve those who might not otherwise be able to afford proper healthcare.

However, you might be surprised to learn how much some physicians enjoy volunteering in free clinics more than they enjoyed their paying job. Not only is it personally rewarding, but doctors say that it's refreshing to not have to deal with the administrative problems or red tape associated with their job. They don't have to be concerned about what an insurance company will pay for or what test to do first to ensure maximum insurance payment.

An additional bonus that volunteering offers for recently retired doctors is the ability to keep abreast of changes in the field. Unfortunately, however, one of the obstacles to retired physicians working in free clinics is that they may need malpractice insurance. If you don't have it, free clinics might turn you away.

Teach

Use your hard-earned wisdom and experience to teach others. Physicians have been teaching in one way or another from their first day of medical school. In practice, physicians are engaged in teaching office staff, patients, medical students on rotation, hospital nursing staffs, etc. It is a part of our blood and relates to our desire to help others and find meaning. Many doctors dream of becoming teachers, and for a lot of them it's a good fit in many ways. Physicians know how to talk to patients about complicated medical concepts in simple terms, and they have had to speak in front of small groups.

In retirement, we can continue that tradition of teaching. Start a free course at your local library or community center. Most medical schools and teaching hospitals welcome retired physicians to participate in clinical teaching on a voluntary basis. You also can teach by writing your own blog online about healthcare issues of importance to you, writing opinion pieces for publication, or volunteer to teach about your own special clinical knowledge to physicians and other healthcare providers in underdeveloped countries.

Despite the financial drawbacks, doctors have a surprisingly strong interest in teaching. In the 2011 Medscape Physician Compensation Report, physicians who wanted to drop clinical medicine chose teaching as one of their top three alternatives. Indeed, teaching is regarded as a relatively stable refuge from the disruptive modern workplace.

Work

Many physicians do not want to completely quit seeing patients in retirement. Part-time salaried positions, working as a locum tenens physician or a per-diem physician can work well for such people. Medical volunteering is another option and discussed also on pages 221 and 230–231. There are many non-clinical options for doctors wishing to work full-time or part-time in retirement. A list of potential non-clinical career options is provided in Table 2.

Sports

Being active physically is important as doctors age. It is the most important component of the Domain of Physical Balance, as defined in Chapter 7. It sustains brain plasticity, keeps muscles and joints supple and flexible, and contributes to glucose metabolism. The endorphin response also sustains positive mood and outlook as we get older. Finding something that you enjoy is critical. Many retired physicians return to the sports and other physical activities they enjoyed in childhood. Still others choose new sporting activities to challenge their personal growth. Doing activities with others not only increases the fun, it keeps you socially connected to others. We have emphasized elsewhere in the book how important connection to others is to the well-being and balance of physicians. So, get out there and have some sports fun!

Hobbies

The demands of practicing medicine make it difficult for many physicians to sustain hobbies. In retirement, however, there is ample time to find new interests and hobbies as well as to return to former interests and hobbies. Activities that build on physicians' creative and musical skills are especially popular. Becoming active in local or national politics, serving on school boards, and volunteering in other ways are considered by many to be hobbies in retirement. Certainly any sporting activities are healthy hobbies to begin or re-engage with in retirement.

Get Healthy

As discussed earlier in this chapter, becoming healthy or healthier should be one of the primary goals of retirement. Doctors know what to do to get healthy. In retirement they finally have the time to do it. Having a health "coach" or personal trainer and a personal physician to help guide you is important to provide personal accountability into your wellness plan.

New Education

Retirement offers innumerable opportunities to challenge your intellect. Look no further than the course catalog of your local community college or university, or the adult education offerings at your local high school. There are almost limitless educational offerings online, many of them available free from well-known universities. Those who choose to launch new businesses or new careers in retirement may need to learn new skills or obtain new certification training in traditional classroom settings or through online learning opportunities. The possibilities are endless. The more you challenge your brain, the less likely you will develop dementia.

A New Career

It's never too late to re-launch in retirement. If you have the passion to do something new, something creative, something to make the world a better place, or to pursue a lifelong business interest, let it rip! Your life experience and wisdom will serve you well.

RETIREMENT CAN BE A TIME FOR NEW BEGINNINGS

Expect to create a new way of living.

No matter where you decide to live (even in the same house you have lived in for 30 years) or what you decide to do, retirement will bring inevitable changes in your way of living. Physicians who are happiest in retirement learn to go with the flow. They don't try to over-plan their day with a frantic list of activities. Take it easy in the first months of retirement. See what wants to happen. Don't be in a big rush to do anything.

If you are observant, listen to your inner voice, and are open to anything new, you will be rewarded with some wonderful new perspectives about how to be happy in retirement.

You may downsize your home.

One kind of new beginning is finding a new home for retirement. Perhaps you have lived in a large house that is now too big a responsibility or expense. Downsizing may offer many advantages. Finding a new environment for retirement living can offer a refreshing, exciting change.

You may find a new community to live in.

Perhaps it is a home in a more desirable part of the country, a smaller place in the mountains with solitude, a big city condo close to the action, or a home closer to your kids and grandchildren. With no work responsibilities to tie you down, you are free in retirement to go wherever your heart and retirement income take you.

You may expand your circle of friends.

With the proper motivation, physicians can seek out and become friends with people from all walks of life—vital, interesting people who share your interests, hobbies, political views, the arts, and outdoor activities as well. Think of new ways to meet new people, both men and women, to expand your network of intimate friends. The larger your community of friends in retirement, the happier you will be. We guarantee that.

You may find new professional contacts and networks.

Now that you have newfound freedom on a daily basis, it is likely that your personal and professional life will expand in new ways. You will meet new people in healthcare, more retired healthcare professionals, and to the extent that you begin to volunteer, undertake new learning and education, or think about starting a new business. You will be flooded with new people to meet. These new people in your life provide new opportunities for networking, expanding your social network for fun and support, and perhaps potential partners or investors for your new business interests.

Physicians of the boomer generation grew up in an era in which social networks did not exist, the Internet did not exist, and we were so focused on moving up the career ladder that we never learned the value of or how to network with other professionals for mutual support, ideas, and growth. We certainly live in a new world today. Everything in business, career development, and even dating is done via Internet searches, networking with like-minded business or healthcare professionals, and using social networks for answering business questions, professional healthcare questions, even for dating and finding life partners.

If you find yourself on the outside of this new world, looking in but not having the computer or social networking skills to participate, find a class, take an online course, hire a teenage to teach you the basics, and welcome a whole new world of fun and adventure!

You may launch a new job, business, or career.

Many of us have harbored a career-long fantasy of doing something entirely unrelated to clinical medicine. Right? But there was never time, you couldn't take the risk, the right opportunity just never seemed to arise.

Retirement provides an antidote to all of those prior concerns. You have all the free time you desire, your finances are now hopefully in excellent shape, your mind is still sharp, and you learn things quickly. Now is the ideal time to launch a new career or a new business. Look around and you will see retired physicians who are now sous chefs, radio/TV commentators, owners of antique stores, vendors of oriental carpets, venture capitalists, real estate agents, ski instructors, to name a few. Often these new business ventures have come directly from childhood hobbies or interests.

Truthfully, it's never too late. All you need is the time and the passion. Get some new education or training to prepare yourself. Do what you love and the money will follow!

FINDING A NEW CALLING

"Calling is the inner urge to give our gifts away. We heed that call when we offer our gifts in service to something we are passionate about in an environment that is consistent with our core values." — Richard Leider

Some physicians decide to engage in a new career or start a new non-healthcare-related business in retirement. Boomer generation physicians are retiring in better health than previous generations of physicians, full of energy and with keen minds. We will see increasing numbers of retired physicians "retool" to enter the workplace doing a variety of new things. Some of these new careers will be in non-clinical aspects of healthcare, and many others will be careers and businesses completely unrelated to medicine and healthcare.

If you are intrigued with this idea, but have no idea of what you want to do or would be good at, don't despair. With some time spent in inner reflection, and if necessary a few sessions with a professional career coach, you will be well on your way to determining your new calling.

The first step is to determine your unique gifts. Calling is intimately related to our unique skills, the things we do well naturally and effortlessly. These are our special gifts. By and large we are born with these gifts rather than acquiring them after years of study or hard work. Make a list of all of your gifts. Get feedback from loved ones and friends who know you well.

Once you have clarified your gifts, consider how you could best "give them away" to benefit others. In so doing, you will have taken a big step toward clarifying your new calling. Table 1 provides some general categories of callings that many physicians adopt in retirement.

TABLE 1. New Callings Retired Physicians Find Enjoyable

The Call to Family
The Call to Spiritual Service
The Call to the Marketplace
The Call to the Professions
The Call to Leadership
The Call to Public Service
The Call to Scholarship
The Call to Nature
The Call of Community

COACHING TIPS FOR FINDING YOUR NEW CALLING

Learn to listen to your inner voice.

Living the stressful, busy lives that practicing physicians lead, there is little down time or quiet time for reflection. Yet it is that kind of quiet reflection that is essential to check in with yourself, to hear and listen to the still, small voice within that represents your wiser self. There are a number of different ways to accomplish this listening within.

Meditation in any form is an excellent approach. Praying and keeping a written journal are two more. Just developing a habit of spending five minutes by yourself in a totally quiet environment upon awakening every day is another easy strategy to enhance self-awareness.

Make an inventory of your unique gifts and talents.

Each of us is born with a unique, innate set of gifts and talents. It is by using those unique gifts and talents that we discover our purpose and our destiny in life. Chances are that during your practice years, you never gave thought to your gifts and talents, you just took them for granted. Physicians without exception are highly talented human beings, capable of accomplishing nearly anything they set out to do because of their rich set of skills, gifts and talents.

Make a list of the things that you do better than anyone you know. Then ask family members, former co-workers, and close friends to tell you what they see as your special gifts and talents. You may be surprised to learn that they see you with skills and talents that you may not appreciate yourself. Once you have clarified your skills and talents, meditate or journal on what kinds of work or new careers would be a good match for you.

Volunteer your time to use your gifts and talents.

Another good way to discover your calling in retirement is to volunteer you time in as many ways and in as many varied settings as possible. Working in new non-medical settings with new people will be an exciting learning experience. You will certainly learn about things you do well despite having no specific education or training. Conversely, you may find that certain tasks or jobs that sounded attractive to you in the beginning of retirement actually turn out to be difficult or even boring in reality.

Return to childhood hobbies and interests.

Chances are that you enjoyed a number of hobbies and had special interests in many things as a kid. Perhaps it was competing in various outdoor sports, collecting stamps, playing the trumpet, building model airplanes or trains, collecting Barbie dolls, collecting all of the Frankie Avalon records, and so on. The fun thing about retirement is that you get the chance to return to your childhood interests if it suits you. And, those childhood interests may offer a clue to your new calling. Think about it.

Develop new skills and knowledge.

One way to know if a new subject of interest to you is really a possible calling is to take a course online or at the local community college to explore that subject in greater depth. Or learn a new physical skill or a new sport to pursue. Some of these explorations eventually lead people to their new calling.

Turn down the volume on your inner critic

Physicians almost always have a stern inner critic. The voice of that inner critic may say things like, " . . . but I'm not smart enough, I'll never be able to learn how to do that, my friends and family wouldn't approve, I can't afford the time it would take, I'm too old for that, and so forth." To prevent that inner critic from running your life, learn how to turn down the volume of that voice. Then go ahead and jump in!

Be willing to take risks and leaps of faith.

Finding a new calling in retirement requires taking risks. Your inner critic will prevent you from taking risks, because the inner critic is afraid of change and afraid of failure. As a retired adult professional, you can simply consider failure a learning experience. Nothing else. If you want the "juice of life," you have to learn to take risks and leaps of faith. Don't obsess or worry, just do it! You may just discover a new calling!

YOU CAN STILL BE PAID AS A RETIRED PHYSICIAN: RE-ENTRY INTO CLINICAL CARE

Retirement from your clinical practice does not have to mean giving up patient care forever, or completely. For some retired physicians, maintaining some relationship to direct patient care is not only a great way to maintain meaning and contribution, it is also a great way to sustain friendships with other practicing physicians, patients, and co-workers. You may be able to stay on in your private practice or clinic as a locum tenens physician or per-diem shift physician. Such part-time work is also an easy and relatively stress-free way to make some extra cash in retirement. These positions are typically non-partnership positions with no benefits, healthcare insurance, or retirement plan contributions. Practices will sometimes put a restriction on the number of years a former partner can remain in such part-time working positions.

One of the obstacles you'll need to consider in physician re-entry is that practices and hospitals might not be able to bear the costs of liability insurance of a physician who hasn't been active for a long time. Returning to the physician's life may seem attractive to a retired doctor, especially if finances are prompting the move back into the workforce. And you'd think it would be an easy transition coming back. Because of his or her ample experience, a retired doctor would need no training— or so it would seem.

In the United States, if you let your license expire and have been inactive for an extended period of time (which, in many states, is only one or two years), re-entry could require new training. This may involve continuing education and passing the Special Purpose Examination (SPEX). This makes sense: if it's been several years since he or she last practiced, a doctor might need to brush up on his or her knowledge and skills. In addition to that, experts in medicine emphasize that technology in the field is continuing to change at an accelerated pace. Doctors may need to prove that they're literate in those technologies and can work with electronic medical records, hospital information systems, voice-activated digital dictation systems, and picture archiving systems (PACS).

Several re-entry programs around the country help get a doctor up to speed. Some states provide the service, while others might require the doctor to pay for it. This is an important matter to look into, as the costs of a re-entry program, which can be upward of $20,000, can be difficult for a retiree.

Teaching Clinical Medicine at Teaching Hospitals

Part-time opportunities for retired, seasoned clinicians to see patients are becoming more commonplace as well in many academic teaching hospitals. Increasing patient case loads, the relatively lower pay scale for full-time faculty physicians, and the high cost of living and housing in the urban environment of most teaching hospitals makes recruiting new full-time faculty more and more challenging. Accordingly, many teaching programs are welcoming retired or part-time private practice physicians to work in salaried, part-time teaching positions. Their responsibilities are primarily in clinician-educator roles. Such physicians are expected to do the bulk of the everyday patient care work and teach and/or supervise medical students and house staff. As with part-time private jobs for retired physicians, these teaching positions are almost always salaried, without benefits.

Locums Tenens Work

Because many retired physicians aren't eager to return to the same schedules, demands, and restrictions of their old job, one popular option is to become a locum tenens doctor. From the Latin for "to hold the place of," locum tenens doctors are those who substitute for others on an as-needed basis. You can get such a job through a staffing agency that will place you with the right healthcare facilities. You could be with one facility for anywhere from a day to a week to a month or longer.

Flexibility is one of the major advantages of this type of job. For instance, part-time locum tenens work is easier to find and often suits the life of a retiree. You'll have some freedom to build your own schedule. Consider, however, that it might require traveling and working off-hours.

Before contacting a staffing agency, check to see whether it pays for travel and accommodations. Of course, this option will also require an active state medical license and, depending on where you practice and if you've been inactive for a while, it may entail the re-entry process discussed above. In fact, depending on the travel required, going into locum tenens work might even necessitate getting licensed in multiple states.

Healthcare Administration

Retired physicians are often very familiar with all of the elements that make a healthcare facility run smoothly, which is why some look into healthcare administration. The job of healthcare administrators is to manage the facility and oversee staff. They are often responsible for developing the rules and regulations of the facility, as well as managing finance, marketing, and human resources issues. Thomas Dolan, president and CEO of the American College of Healthcare Executives, says that knowing how medicine is delivered and having clinical experience helps in becoming an administrator (personal communication).

Not all retired doctors will have a desire to become an administrator. Although their clinical patient care experience will certainly help, it takes a different set of skills to manage a facility than to practice medicine. "The real challenge" for such a transition, says Dolan, "is for those doctors who are not trained in business." Today, many administrators hold specialized degrees in healthcare administration, nursing administration, or business administration. And, if you're interested in nursing home administration, this will require getting licensed. The good news is that, according to the U.S. Department of Labor, the demand for healthcare administrators is on the rise.

Telemedicine

If you have computer literacy, a phone, and a reliable Internet connection, you might be able to find part-time or full-time work from home helping to treat patients online. Services like AmeriDoc.com like to argue that virtual doctor consultations are an efficient alternative that can also alleviate demands on doctors' offices. They contend on their website (www.AmeriDoc.com) that, as one of their telemedicine doctors, you can diagnose minor medical problems and even prescribe non-controlled medications (as opposed to controlled medications, which are more tightly regulated).

Telemedicine can be delivered to patients 24 hours a day, seven days a week, and this can be accomplished from any geographic location. Because of this, physicians have the ability to participate in medical care when they are at great geographic separation between patient and provider.

There's a demand for doctors willing to participate in telemedicine environment. At the present time and in the foreseeable future, there is a shortage of providers; thus, telemedicine is able to solve this problem as it now makes it possible for physicians to practice medicine regardless of where they live and if they wish to have limited hours of practice.

For a list of the top 10 companies in telemedicine, visit www.bccresearch.com/market-research/healthcare/telemedicine-top-ten-companies-hlc130a.html

For the doctor who wishes to consider staying involved in healthcare, who wants to work a limited schedule, and who is comfortable not being face to face with the patient, telemedicine may be a viable option.

CLINICAL VOLUNTEERING AS A RETIRED PHYSICIAN

Another option for retired physicians who wish to maintain some activity in clinical medicine is to find an opportunity to perform unpaid volunteer patient care services.

There are numerous opportunities for physician volunteering in your local community if you seek them out. These may include working in medical clinics for the underserved population, being a team physician for local high school teams, teaching residents and medical students at your nearest medical school or affiliated teaching hospital, seeing the world as a volunteer physician for international care agencies such as The Good Ship Hope, and the numerous church-based healthcare missions throughout the underdeveloped world. Some physicians enjoy volunteering for the Red Cross and other international aid agencies at the time of world natural disasters such as a major earthquake, hurricane, or tsunami.

To participate in medical volunteering, you will of course need to maintain your state medical license and maintain specialty board certification if that is important to the kind of volunteering you prefer. Doing both requires you to maintain your knowledge and skill set by taking continuing medical education courses in your field of volunteering.

NON-CLINICAL CAREER OPTIONS
FOR THE RETIRED PHYSICIAN

You may decide that you don't really want to become engaged in direct patient care, but would like to stay involved in healthcare in some productive, meaningful way that takes advantage of your many years of clinical practice experience. Physicians are increasingly turning to non-clinical careers to meet this need as an alternative to direct patient care, in addition to direct patient care, or in retirement as a way to stay engaged in the healthcare industry.

While the details of all possible non-clinical careers are beyond the scope of this book, you will find a list of popular non-clinical options for physicians at any stage of their career in Table 2. Some of these non-clinical options can be entered directly from practice. Others may require additional training, education, or certification.

Those who are interested in learning more about specific career opportunities in any of these fields can find such information in the books and conferences produced by SEAK, Inc. (www.seak.com).

TABLE 2. A List of Potential Non-Clinical Careers for Physicians

Pharma Medical Science Liaisons
Medical Informatics Consultant to Healthcare Organizations
Federal Government Disability Insurance Industry
Venture Capital Expert Witness Work
Entrepreneur Disability and File Review
Inventor Television Journalism
Medical Communications/Advertising Medical Writing
Health Insurance Consultant Consulting Firms
Independent Medical Examinations Public Health Work
Consulting Firms Wellness Coaching
Television Journalism Healthcare Liaison
Medical Administration Career or Life Coaching
Public Health Medical Writing

Consulting

A great way to continue contributing your expertise to the healthcare community while maintaining a semi-retired lifestyle is to become a consultant.

Your consulting could go beyond medicine, as well. Some healthcare facilities take on medical consultants to help plan new facilities. They may take on consulting physicians to take the burden of this planning off their practicing physicians who need time to focus on patients. And you don't necessarily have to become a consultant for a healthcare facility. Because medical consultants are needed in so many fields, you have a lot of options.

For instance, medical device manufacturers often require medical consultants for their advice on product and liability issues. Law firms often seek medical consultants for expertise or testimony in malpractice cases. Others take on consultants to verify the medical accuracy of their publications or advertisements. Consider government organizations such as the Social Security Administration, state health systems, and insurance companies, all of which need medical consultants to help evaluate disability claims.

Writing and Editing

Do you enjoy keeping a journal? Do you ever notice egregious mistakes and misinformation about medicine floating around in popular publications? If you have decent writing skills and a sense of proper grammar, you might enjoy writing and editing.

It can be the perfect opportunity for retired physicians who simply prefer staying within the comfort of their home while making some extra money. The amount of medical information online has exploded, and more and more people like to look up their own symptoms on the Internet before even calling the doctor. Web sites that want to provide reliable information might offer freelance work for a retired physician to write online articles or examine other articles for accuracy. This type of work obviously requires word processing computer literacy.

With their new freedom, other retired physicians choose to flex their more creative writing muscles. Some choose to incorporate their expertise in writing medical suspense novels, for instance. If you can find a publisher for the kind of writing you'd be passionate about, this might be the ideal second career for you.

Writing as a freelance contributor to trade journals and magazines is another option for physician writers. The work tends to be somewhat sporadic and less-predictable than working for a medical communications company. However if income is not a significant motivator, freelance writing can be very satisfying.

Finally, writing and publishing your own blog online is the easiest solution for physician writers who are not interesting in a predictable income, and who do not cherish the thought of having publication deadlines to deal with. Blogs offer the opportunity for you to write about topics that interest you, that you are passionate about, and topics about which you are well informed.

Medical writing is a competitive industry. It is unlikely that you will be able to replace your clinical practice income. However salaries in the six figures are not unusual for experienced physician writers in industry. Corporate entities employing physicians as writers typically require the submission of a portfolio of your writing for them to evaluate prior to offering an interview.

AN OLD DOC'S REFLECTIONS ON RETIREMENT
By Peter S. Moskowitz, MD

At the end of my first year of retirement, I sat down to reflect on my experiences and how they compared with my expectations. What follows is a short commentary of how things unfolded. I hope it will provide inspiration to others who are about to retire, valued wisdom from my personal experience, and encouragement to dive into retirement yourself.

It is odd the way my first year of retirement has unfolded. A time that I looked forward to and worked so hard for has been full of surprises.

I worried that I would miss the ebb and flow of clinical practice and the ego satisfaction of being a physician. I have seen that happen so many times to physicians who had no identity or interests outside of clinical medicine. Playing golf every day can get boring very quickly. I played a total of two rounds of golf in my first year of retirement.

Truthfully, I have not for one minute missed my old life or practice. Perhaps that is a testament to the years of preparation I made to be ready. Preparation to keep myself engaged in life, to be more physically healthy, to stay actively connected to others, to keep learning, and to have meaningful non-clinical work (my physician coaching practice).

I worried that I would be bored, with not enough to do to keep my mind active, that I would have to find multiple new things to keep myself busy all day long. Instead, I have come to realize that doing less is much better than doing more.

I worried I would become slovenly and sleep until noon. I haven't. I still get up at 6 a.m. most days, but now I wake up well rested. The secret: I now go to bed earlier (10 p.m.) than in the past. I get 8 hours of sleep every night. I wake up refreshed and full of energy to start a new day. I do my exercise first thing in the morning when I have the energy and the mindset to get it done.

I discovered that in retirement, you get to have the pleasure of becoming friends with yourself once again. One needs quiet time alone to best renew that friendship. Only in quiet solitude have I come to realize just how frenetic and crazy my life has been day in and day out, for decades. No way to hear my own inner voice of wisdom. Today I hear that voice regularly. I am comfortable in my own skin.

Certainly I have found new challenges and things to do that are fun. I am learning to enjoy gourmet cooking and the pleasure it brings to others. I am actually good at something I knew absolutely nothing about 1 year ago. I have taken several courses at Stanford, including most recently, The Psychology of Happiness. I enjoy breakfasts and lunches with old retired physician friends. We talk mostly about everything except medicine. What a pleasure.

I have committed myself to improving my own wellness by eating a more healthy diet in quality and quantity, and increasing my physical activity to include weight training for an hour three times a week with the help of a personal trainer. I have become fit, lost 17 pounds, and gained self-esteem and energy. I am much more relaxed and happy.

Several of my goals for the first year of retirement are not yet completed, but I am already seeing the rewards. I vowed to re-organize my home office files, discard years of outdated paperwork and records, and clean out my closet and attic of old and/or unused "stuff" and clothing. I'm nearly done with that. To my surprise, that has had the unexpected effect of increasing my sense of well-being, order, and calmness.

Perhaps the most important lessons of my first year of retirement have been learning the value of simplification, the value of "doing" less and "being" more, the joys of connecting and sharing myself more with others, challenging myself a bit to learn new things, and yet not setting too many expectations for myself.

In all, it has been a very good year.

PUTTING IT ALL TOGETHER: THE KEYS TO SUCCESS IN RETIREMENT

We hope that this chapter has provided you with confidence that you will be able to enter retirement not only well prepared for success, but with many strategies to keep you healthy, happy, and full of ideas for a retirement rich in meaning, contribution, and intellectual stimulation.

As we see it, the keys to success in retirement revolve around a thoughtful plan to keep yourself healthy, a well-planned and executed financial and income plan, judicious spending, values-based use of your time and money, keeping your mind alive, giving away your skills and experience to the benefit of others, and saving daily time for fun!

Afterword

THERE IS NOTHING QUITE LIKE BEING A DOCTOR, whatever career stage you are in. In every stage you have a unique and special opportunity to be of great service to your patients. Most of us feel an enormous sense of satisfaction and enjoyment from this wonderful profession.

To help you navigate the many challenges of your profession, we dissected a medical career into three stages: The Early-Career Physician, The Mid-Career Physician, and the Late-Career Physician. Our goal was to present to you a "go-to" resource on career and business management highlighting the unique issues, concerns, and challenges you'll have during the three very different stages of your career. We outlined the skills you'll need to navigate the waters from the beginning of your career to its successful end.

We provided Early-Career Physicians with a rationale for choosing a field of specialization, an understanding of modern career theory to assist them in career self-management, and strategies for planning career transitions. The importance of finding a balance between a doctor's professional life and his or her personal life and how to become skilled at doing so was discussed in detail. How well you maintain this balance will ultimately determine not only your success, but also your personal health and happiness. All of these topics and strategies are rarely discussed during medical training.

Successful doctors must also have an understanding of the business aspects of medical practice. We believe that by having good advisors, by saving and investing at the beginning and middle of your career, and having appropriate mechanisms to protect your practice and your estate, you can reach the end of medical practice and begin retirement with confidence and ample financial resources. The goal is to live out the remaining years of your life in a lifestyle that does not require you to change your standard of living.

In our view, the greatest challenges for the Late-Career Physician revolve around successfully exiting from clinical practice, selling the practice, and planning for a secure, exciting, and meaningful life after retirement. We provided roadmaps to successfully accomplish all of these important goals.

Our hope is that, with this book as your guide, you will gain the foundations necessary to have the medical practice, the medical career, and the retirement of your dreams.

Best wishes navigating your medical career, enjoying good health and balance, and forging a happy and meaningful retirement.

NEIL H. BAUM, MD
JOEL M. BLAU, CFP®
PETER S. MOSKOWITZ, MD
RONALD J. PAPROCKI, CFP®, JD

INDEX

Workplace
    absences, 150
    relationship conflicts, 87
Work relative value units (wRVUs), 36
Writing/editing, expertise, 226–227

Y

Younger physicians, practice initiation/
    building, 179–180